Cancer Prevention

A Mistake in the Lifeline - Rectified

Dr. Sasi Shanmugam Senga

KCF Press
Boston • London
Newark, DE 19713, USA

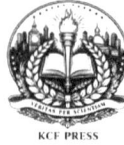

Cancer Prevention

A Mistake in the Lifeline - Rectified

© 2021 Sasi Shanmugam Senga

Published by KCF Press
Boston • London
KCF Press is a nonprofit publishing imprint.

This work was independently authored and editorially reviewed prior to publication.

First published 2021
ISBN 978-0-6489285-0-8
Library of Congress Control Number (LCCN): 2021905482

This book is intended for informational and conceptual purposes only and does not constitute medical advice. It should not be used as a substitute for professional medical judgment, diagnosis, or treatment.

Contents

Chapter 14
Precision Prevention of Cervical Cancer

Chapter 15
Precision Prevention of Prostate Cancer

Chapter 16
Precision Prevention: Environmental Risk Factors

Chapter 17
Precision Prevention: Infections Beyond HPV and
Hepatitis

Chapter 18
Early Symptoms People Ignore

Final Interlude
What I Tell My Own Family

Epilogue
Do Not Surrender These Years to the Crab

Appendix
What to Do

References
Index

About the Author

Dr. Sasi Shanmugam Senga is a neurosurgical oncologist with a Master's degree in Neuroscience and a Master's degree in Cancer and Therapeutics. He is a UK Commonwealth Scholar, an Oxford Clarendon Scholar, and a recipient of the Harvard Excellence Award.

He has served as a lecturer in Medicine at the University of Oxford and the University of Buckingham, and as Programme Director in Molecular Genetics and Ethics at Stanford University. He has also contributed to international policy and research discussions as a panellist for *The Economist* think tanks.

In parallel with his academic work, he is involved in the evaluation of global higher-education systems and contributes annually to the QS World University Rankings for top universities worldwide.

He is an Ambassador and active member of leading international cancer organisations, including the European Association for Cancer Research, the European Society for Medical Oncology, the American Association for Cancer Research, and the American Society of Clinical Oncology.

Dr. Senga is the author of a Royal Society–top-cited research article, *Hallmarks of Cancer: The New Testament*. His work lies at the intersection of cancer biology, ageing, neuroscience, ethics, and the limits of medical intervention.

In memory of Kalavathi

mother of the author,
whose life and death shaped the author's path toward
contributing, in however small a way, to the benefit of
humankind.

Prologue

I was holding a syringe in my hand.

It was meant to raise my mother's white blood cell count after chemotherapy. I had given this injection many times before, to strangers, to patients whose names sometimes faded from memory by morning.

This time was different.

My mother was dying of metastatic cancer.

I prepared the dose carefully. My hands did not shake. That, more than anything, unsettled me.

None of it altered the essential fact that the disease was advancing.

Later that evening, I found myself reading a blog written by a father in the United States. His daughter had metastatic triple-negative breast cancer. He described long drives to distant specialists, the careful hope invested in each cycle of treatment.

On the drive home after chemotherapy, she vomited into a bag while he kept the car moving, mile after mile.

I recognised the scene immediately.

Near the end of the post, he wrote something that unsettled me: that those who have lost loved ones to cancer must enter research themselves, because only then would meaningful change occur.

It was an accusation I could not dismiss.

I had entered medicine because I loved science. More truthfully, I had entered it because I wanted to fight cancer.

Somewhere along the long arc of training, I drifted, drawn toward surgery, toward problems that could be confronted decisively, toward outcomes that felt immediate.

Oncology unsettled me.

During my rotations, I watched patients arrive at clinics carrying bottles of wine, speaking softly about putting their affairs in order, planning final journeys, saying careful goodbyes. The oncologist's role, so vital, so humane, often became one of negotiation rather than rescue.

Saving life gave way to preserving its quality.

At the time, I mistook this for failure.

Only later did I understand how flawed that belief was, and how dangerous. Cancer does not yield to heroics alone. It yields to understanding.

After my mother died, I chose a path that tried to reconcile these tensions. I trained as a neurosurgical oncologist, holding on to surgery while committing myself fully to cancer research.

I no longer remember the name of the father who wrote that blog, nor the platform on which I read it. But his words accomplished what lectures and textbooks had not: they returned me to my original purpose.

Cancer exposes an imbalance we rarely acknowledge.

A person diagnosed with the disease is expected to make life-altering decisions while knowing almost nothing about what is unfolding inside their own body. Meanwhile, the clinician holds years, sometimes decades, of specialised knowledge.

This asymmetry leaves patients vulnerable at the very moment they most need agency.

Your body is your most valuable possession. It is the instrument through which every experience of living occurs. To surrender decisions about it without understanding is not inevitable; it is a failure of communication.

This book was born from that realisation.

Cancer is often described as bad luck.
A random mutation.
A roll of the dice.

Chance plays a role.

But a growing body of evidence suggests that many cancers are strongly influenced by lifestyle and environmental choices.

Recognising this does not assign blame.
It restores agency.

This book is about how that realisation changed my life, and why it may change yours.

A Note to the Reader

The language used in this book is intentionally accessible. Its purpose is to increase public understanding of cancer prevention and risk, not to engage in technical debate. Readers seeking a more specialised, research-focused discussion may refer to my peer-reviewed work with the Royal Society (Senga et al., 2021), which was written for a scientific audience.

Cancer is often described as a matter of bad luck. While chance plays a role, a growing body of evidence suggests that many cancers are strongly influenced by lifestyle and environmental choices. Recognising this does not assign blame, it restores agency.

Chapter 1

Cancer: An Ancient Disease in a Modern World

The Bone

The bone lay in the dust longer than anyone alive had existed.

It was small enough to be overlooked, a fragment of a foot, weathered smooth by time, lifted carefully from the earth at the Cradle of Humankind, northwest of Johannesburg. No ornamentation. No ceremony. Just calcium, mineral, and absence.

Under the African sun, it appeared ordinary.

Only later, under magnification, did its silence begin to speak.

The surface was irregular. The architecture distorted. Growth where growth did not belong. The kind of pattern that, once learned, cannot be unseen.

This individual had lived 1.8 million years ago.

There were no factories.
No cigarettes.
No artificial light bleeding into night.

Yet the bone bore the unmistakable signature
of osteosarcoma, an aggressive cancer of bone (Odes EJ et
al., 2016).

Cancer had not arrived with modern life.

It had been waiting.

An Ancient Companion

Cancer is often described as a disease of modernity. The
evidence tells a different story.

It is not confined to humans.

In 1999, Dr. Bruce Rothschild identified evidence of
metastatic cancer in dinosaur fossils (Rothschild et al.,
1999). In 2019, German researchers discovered a
malignant bone tumour in a 240-million-year-old stem
turtle fossil.

Cancer predates civilisation.
It predates industry.
It predates humanity itself.

The fossilised hominin foot from South Africa was not an anomaly. It was part of a much older pattern, genetic vulnerabilities embedded deep within multicellular life.

Cancer, it seems, is an ancient companion.

Cancer in the Dead Who Would Not Decay

Human remains have preserved further evidence.

A 2003 study of Egyptian mummies revealed a case of rectal cancer (Zimmerman et al., 2003). Even more revealing were discoveries from naturally mummified bodies preserved in church crypts in Hungary, used between 1731 and 1838.

Pine shavings placed in coffins and stable temperatures near 8°C created ideal conditions for preservation. Genetic analysis of these remains uncovered mutations in the adenomatous polyposis coli (APC) gene, mutations still commonly observed in colorectal cancer today (Feldman et al., 2016).

These findings force an uncomfortable question:

If cancer existed long before industrialisation, why does it appear so common now?

One explanation is visibility: ancient cancers are harder to detect.

Another is longevity: people now live long enough for cancer to emerge.

But a third possibility is more unsettling.

While cancer is ancient, its incidence has accelerated, shaped by modern environments, behaviours, and exposures.

From Curse to Cause

Early civilisations recognised cancer, though they struggled to explain it.

The Edwin Smith Papyrus (c. 3000 BC) describes breast cancer (Breasted, 1930). The Ebers Papyrus (c. 1500 BC) documents tumours of the skin, uterus, and other organs (Ebbell, 1937). Cancer was often regarded as a curse, mysterious, incurable, beyond human control.

Greek medicine replaced myth with theory.

Hippocrates coined the term *carcinos*, likening invasive tumours to a crab. He proposed that cancer arose from an excess of black bile, a theory later expanded by Galen, physician to Emperor Marcus Aurelius (Galen, Linacre and Siberch, 1521).

The idea endured for centuries.

Until the 16th century, when anatomist Andreas Vesalius demonstrated, through dissection, that black bile did not exist (Vesalius, 1543).

The theory collapsed.

Cancer remained.

The Environment Enters the Story

A decisive shift occurred with Paracelsus, who observed arsenic and sulphur deposits in the blood of mine workers and linked these exposures to cancer, laying the foundation for occupational oncology.

By the 18th century, the evidence sharpened:

- In 1761, John Hill linked snuff use to cancer (*Cautions against the Immoderate Use of Snuff*).
- In 1775, Sir Percival Pott identified scrotal cancer among chimney sweeps exposed to soot, the first clear demonstration of cancer as an occupational disease.

Industrialisation intensified risk.

In 1856, William Henry Perkin synthesised aniline dye. By 1895, surgeon Ludwig Rehn observed high rates of bladder cancer among dye factory workers, linking aniline exposure to malignancy.

Progress, it seemed, carried a biological cost.

Cancer at the Cellular Level

In 1914, Theodor Boveri proposed that abnormal segregation of chromosomes during cell division could initiate tumour formation.

Today, this idea has matured into a sophisticated understanding of cancer as a disease of genetic instability and cellular diversity. Even a single tumour may contain multiple genetically distinct populations, a phenomenon known as intratumoral heterogeneity.

Cancer is not one enemy.

It is many.

What Cancer Is

Only now can we name it clearly.

Cancer is not a single disease.
It is a heterogeneous group of disorders united by one defining failure: the inability of cells to obey the body's regulatory signals.

Normal cells divide, mature, and die in response to precise instructions. Cancer cells ignore those instructions. The result is uncontrolled growth, invasion of surrounding tissue, and, often, spread to distant organs.

Understanding this failure is essential.
So is recognising its context.

From Inevitability to Influence

Our understanding of cancer has progressed, from curses to chromosomes, from superstition to cell biology. Yet despite extraordinary advances in treatment, one challenge remains unresolved: how to destroy cancer without destroying the life it inhabits.

This reality makes prevention not secondary, but central.

If cancer were purely a matter of fate, prevention would be futile. History tells a different story. While genetic susceptibility is ancient, many drivers of cancer, environmental toxins, dietary patterns, physical inactivity, circadian disruption, chronic inflammation, are distinctly modern.

Cancer may not always be preventable.

But it is often influenceable.

And influence begins with understanding.

Chapter 2

You Are What You Eat

The table was unremarkable.

A bowl of Greek yogurt, thick and faintly sour.
A glass of buttermilk, cool against the palm.
A small dish of Korean kimchi, its fermented sharpness
rising before the first bite.

There was nothing indulgent about the meal. No excess.
No performance. Just food prepared the way humans have
prepared food for most of their history, by allowing time,
microbes, and chemistry to do their work.

What struck me was not the simplicity, but what followed.

Within minutes of eating, trillions of microorganisms would
respond. Some would awaken, others would multiply, and
still others would begin producing molecules that never
appear on nutrition labels, short-chain fatty acids, immune-
modulating metabolites, signalling compounds that would
enter the bloodstream and travel to distant organs.

The body would register none of this consciously.
No sensation. No signal. No awareness.

Yet the effects would be real.

Only later did I learn how to describe what was happening.

It was not digestion alone.
It was dialogue.

Every meal, whether we notice it or not, initiates a conversation between what we eat and the microscopic life that inhabits us. Over time, that conversation shapes inflammation, immunity, metabolism, and, increasingly clearly, cancer risk.

2.1 The Microbiome: An Overlooked Ally in Cancer Prevention

Humans are not composed solely of human cells.

We are ecosystems.

The microbial cells that inhabit our bodies, collectively known as the microbiome, outnumber our own cells many times over. The microbial metagenome exceeds the human genome by at least a hundredfold (Huttenhower et al., 2012).

These microorganisms are not passive passengers. They are active participants in metabolism, immunity, and health.

Microbes have existed on Earth for approximately 3.25 billion years (Allwood et al., 2006). Multicellular life emerged much later, around 1.25 billion years ago

(Butterfield, Knoll, and Swett, 1990). It is therefore unavoidable that evolution was shaped not in isolation, but in constant interaction with microbes. Modern biology confirms this relationship: microorganisms regulate host metabolism, immune responses, and cellular homeostasis (Bäckhed et al., 2005).

Strikingly, nearly half of the metabolites detected in human plasma are derived from microbial activity (Martin et al., 2007). For this reason, the microbiome has been described as the "forgotten organ." Unlike our genetic code, however, this organ is not fixed. It responds rapidly to diet, environment, medications, and lifestyle.

This plasticity makes the microbiome a compelling target, not for curing cancer, but for reducing risk.

2.2 Probiotics: Lessons from History and Biology

At the turn of the 20th century, Nobel laureate Elie Metchnikoff became fascinated by longevity. In his book *The Prolongation of Life* (1900), he described individuals who reportedly lived well beyond a century, including Saint Mungo, the agriculturist Pierre Zortay, and a Norwegian named Drakenburg. While such ages invite scepticism, Metchnikoff focused less on numbers and more on patterns.

He observed that populations consuming fermented milk appeared to enjoy better health and longer lives. Metchnikoff proposed that fermented foods promoted a favourable microbial environment in the gut. He practiced what he preached, consuming soured milk daily for years, and reporting personal satisfaction with the results.

More than a century later, science has refined, but not dismissed, his intuition.

How Probiotics May Reduce Cancer Risk

Probiotics do not act through a single mechanism. Their effects are strain-specific, context-dependent, and cumulative.

1. Suppression of Pathogenic Bacteria

Probiotics can limit colonisation by harmful microbes through several mechanisms: competition for nutrients, production of antimicrobial compounds, and physical aggregation that prevents pathogen attachment. Experimental and clinical studies have demonstrated probiotic-mediated suppression of *Staphylococcus aureus* and *Clostridium difficile* infections (Piewngam et al., 2018; Mills et al., 2018).

By reducing chronic inflammation and exposure to microbial toxins, this suppression may indirectly lower cancer-promoting signals in the host.

2. Immune Modulation and Surveillance

Probiotics interact closely with the immune system. Fermented milk consumption has been shown to enhance humoral immunity, including significant increases in serum immunoglobulin A (IgA) levels (Link-Amster et al., 1994).

This immune crosstalk may strengthen immunosurveillance, the process by which the immune system identifies and eliminates cells undergoing malignant transformation. While immunosurveillance is not infallible, its impairment is a recognised feature of cancer development.

3. Vaginal Microbiome, HPV, and Cervical Cancer

The relationship between microbiota and cancer risk is particularly well illustrated in cervical cancer.

More than 85% of human papillomavirus (HPV) infections are cleared spontaneously by the immune system (Shulzhenko et al., 2014). Why, then, do the remaining infections persist and progress to cervical neoplasia?

A growing body of evidence points to vaginal microbiome dysbiosis.

In healthy individuals, the vaginal microbiome is dominated by *Lactobacillus* species (Martin and Marrazzo,

2016). These bacteria maintain an acidic environment (pH < 4.5) through lactic acid production, creating a barrier against pathogens. *Lactobacillus* species inhibit viruses such as herpes simplex virus (Conti et al., 2009), human immunodeficiency virus (Tyssen et al., 2018), *Neisseria gonorrhoeae* (Graver and Wade, 2011), and *Escherichia coli* (Cadieux et al., 2009).

Loss of *Lactobacillus* dominance has been associated with increased acquisition of HPV and reduced viral clearance (Łaniewski et al., 2018). Increased vaginal microbial diversity, often considered beneficial elsewhere in the body, correlates strongly with the severity of cervical neoplasia (Mitra et al., 2015; Łaniewski et al., 2018).

Importantly, intervention studies offer cautious optimism. Women with HPV-positive low-grade squamous intraepithelial lesions who consumed a probiotic drink daily for six months demonstrated improved HPV clearance and regression of cytological abnormalities (Verhoeven et al., 2013).

A Measured Conclusion

Probiotics are not cures. They are not substitutes for screening, vaccination, or medical care. But as part of a broader lifestyle strategy, they may support microbial balance, immune competence, and cancer risk reduction.

Caution is essential. Certain bacterial strains, such as genotoxic *pks+ Escherichia coli*, are harmful and should never be present in probiotic formulations. While such strains are uncommon in commercial probiotics, informed selection matters, particularly for individuals with immunosuppression or other predisposing conditions.

Cancer prevention rarely hinges on a single choice. It emerges from patterns repeated daily, what we eat, how we live, and how we coexist with the unseen organisms that share our bodies.

Food, in this sense, is not merely nourishment.
It is biological instruction.

Chapter 3

When Life Loses Its Rhythm

The alarm rings long before dawn.

Outside, the street is silent. Curtains are drawn tight against the night, but inside the room a blue glow already fills the air. A phone lights up first, then a laptop. Coffee brews. Breakfast is skipped. There is no hunger yet, only urgency.

By the time the sun rises, the body has already been awake for hours.

Across the city, a nurse steps out of a hospital at the end of a night shift. The light feels wrong, too bright, too sudden. Sleep will come later, fragmented and shallow, interrupted by traffic, by daylight, by a world that insists it is time to be awake.

At an airport, a flight attendant crosses time zones faster than the body can follow. Morning becomes night. Night becomes afternoon. Meals arrive without hunger. Sleep comes without rest.

None of this feels dangerous.

It feels normal. Productive. Necessary.

The body does not protest. Not immediately.

It adapts. It compensates. It waits.

Years later, when disease finally appears, it will not announce its origin. It will not say: this began when night became day, when meals lost their hour, when sleep became negotiable.

It will simply arrive.

At dawn, birds begin to sing. Seasons arrive and depart with remarkable regularity. Across nature, timing is not incidental, it is essential.

Humans, however, are increasingly out of step.

We possess an internal timing system known as the circadian rhythm, a biological clock that governs sleep and wakefulness, metabolism, hormone secretion, immune activity, and cellular repair. When this rhythm is chronically disrupted, the consequences extend far beyond fatigue. Mounting evidence suggests that disturbance of the circadian rhythm can contribute to tumourigenesis, the process by which normal cells become cancerous.

3.1 The Circadian Clock

The circadian clock is an autonomous biological oscillator that operates on an approximately 24-hour cycle. While it is self-sustaining, it remains highly responsive to environmental cues such as light exposure, temperature, feeding patterns, and periods of fasting.

The master clock resides in a small region of the brain known as the suprachiasmatic nucleus (SCN), located in the hypothalamus. This central clock synchronises a network of peripheral clocks present in nearly every tissue of the body. Like the interlocking gears of a mechanical watch, communication between the central and peripheral clocks maintains physiological harmony, what biologists refer to as homeostasis.

One of the most important outputs of the circadian system is melatonin, a hormone primarily secreted by the pineal gland. Melatonin levels rise in darkness and fall with light exposure. Prolonged exposure to artificial light after sunset, particularly from mobile phones, tablets, and laptops, suppresses melatonin secretion.

This suppression matters. Beyond regulating sleep, melatonin has antioxidant properties and has been implicated in pathways that inhibit cancer development. Observational studies have linked exposure to artificial light at night with an increased risk of breast cancer (Yang et al., 2014).

Shift Work, Sleep Loss, and Cancer Risk

The health effects of circadian disruption are perhaps most clearly observed in populations whose work requires persistent misalignment with natural light–dark cycles.

The landmark Nurses' Health Study revealed that nurses who worked three or more night shifts per week for at least fifteen years had a significantly increased risk of developing colorectal cancer (Schernhammer et al., 2003). Subsequent studies have demonstrated that night-shift work is associated with elevated inflammatory markers, suggesting a biological mechanism linking circadian disruption to cancer-promoting inflammation (Amano et al., 2018).

Flight attendants represent another high-risk group. Frequent travel across time zones, irregular sleep schedules, and repeated circadian misalignment have been associated with increased cancer risk in multiple studies, including the Harvard Flight Attendant Health Study (McNeely et al., 2018; Grajewski et al., 2016).

These findings are not indictments of professions, they are warnings about biology.

Eating Time Matters as Much as Eating Choices

Circadian rhythms do not respond to light alone. Food timing is a powerful synchroniser of peripheral clocks, particularly in the liver and metabolic tissues.

Hormones such as ghrelin, which regulates appetite, and leptin, which signals satiety, follow circadian patterns. Eating late at night disrupts these hormonal rhythms and has been linked to weight gain and obesity (Garaulet et al., 2014). Obesity itself is a well-established risk factor for multiple cancers.

Beyond weight, food timing directly influences gene expression. Studies have shown that irregular eating patterns can alter the expression of genes responsible for maintaining circadian rhythm, particularly in the liver (Damiola et al., 2000).

Large population studies support these molecular findings. The French NutriNet-Santé cohort, which followed over 41,000 adults, reported that late evening meals were associated with circadian disruption and a higher propensity for cancer development (Srour et al., 2018).

Circadian rhythm and Immune defense

The immune system does not operate uniformly throughout the day. Its activity follows circadian oscillations, optimising surveillance and response at specific times.

The importance of immune function in cancer prevention is underscored by the Nobel Prize–winning work of James P. Allison and Tasuku Honjo, whose discoveries transformed cancer immunotherapy. Yet immune competence is diminished when circadian rhythms are disrupted. Experimental studies demonstrate that circadian misalignment impairs immune signalling and reduces the body's ability to identify and eliminate emerging cancer cells (Gibbs et al., 2014).

Circadian disruption may therefore promote cancer both directly, by altering cell cycle control, and indirectly, through inflammation, metabolic dysfunction, obesity, and immune suppression.

Restoring the Rhythm

The circadian clock is remarkably resilient. Unlike genetic mutations, it can be retrained.

Regular sleep schedules, exposure to natural daylight, avoidance of bright screens late at night, consistent meal timing, and prioritisation of sleep quality all help restore circadian alignment. These habits are not merely lifestyle preferences, they are biological signals.

Cancer prevention does not rely on perfection. It relies on patterns.

By supporting the rhythm of life, day and night, fasting and feeding, activity and rest, we strengthen one of the most ancient protective systems encoded within us.

Chapter 4

A Sweet Way to Become Fat

The vending machine hummed softly at the end of the hospital corridor.

Its glass front glowed in the late afternoon light, rows of chocolate bars and sugared drinks arranged with quiet efficiency. A young man stood in front of it, scrolling through his phone with one hand while feeding coins into the slot with the other. He hesitated only briefly before pressing the button.

No one passing him would have thought twice.

He was not visibly overweight. There was no excess, no indulgence, no spectacle. Just sugar, easily obtained, quietly consumed.

What his body would do with it, however, was already decided.

Within minutes, glucose would surge into his bloodstream. Insulin would rise in response. Energy not immediately required would be diverted, efficiently, invisibly, into storage. Not into muscle. Not into function. But into adipose tissue, where it would wait: metabolically active, hormonally influential, and anything but inert.

This is how modern disease begins.
Not with indulgence, but with normality.

A sweet tooth does more than damage teeth.
Over time, it reshapes metabolism, hormones, and risk.

From Survival to Surplus

As humans transitioned from the Palaeolithic era to the modern age, our relationship with food changed profoundly. For most of human history, calories were scarce and physically costly to obtain. The agricultural revolution introduced refined carbohydrates; industrialisation made them abundant; modern life removed the physical effort once required to access them.

Today, calorie-dense foods are readily available, while physical activity has steadily declined.

The result is a persistent imbalance between energy intake and energy expenditure. Excess energy is stored as fat, primarily within adipose tissue. This storage is not passive. Adipose tissue is biologically active and unevenly distributed, patterns shaped by genetics, sex, and hormones.

Men tend to accumulate fat around the abdomen.
Women more commonly store fat in the hips, thighs, and buttocks.

These patterns matter biologically, not cosmetically.

Measuring Obesity: Beyond the Scale

One commonly used marker of obesity is body mass index (BMI), calculated as weight in kilograms divided by height in meters squared (kg/m²). According to the World Health Organisation, a BMI between 18.5 and 24.9 is considered healthy (WHO, 2017).

BMI, however, is an imperfect measure.

Waist circumference better reflects visceral fat, the metabolically active fat surrounding internal organs. Cut-off values associated with increased health risk are approximately:

- 94 cm for Western men
- 90 cm for Asian men
- 80 cm for women

For a meaningful assessment of obesity-related risk, both BMI and waist circumference must be considered.

4.1 Adult Weight Gain and Cancer Risk

The most compelling evidence linking obesity to cancer does not come from childhood weight, but from adult weight gain, the gradual accumulation of excess fat during adulthood.

Adult weight gain more accurately reflects increases in adipose tissue rather than lean mass. It is this tissue that alters biological signalling in ways that promote carcinogenesis.

Adipose tissue secretes pro-inflammatory cytokines, establishing a state of chronic low-grade inflammation. It also influences circulating levels of oestrogen and insulin, often leading to insulin resistance.

Together, these changes create a biological environment that quietly favours cancer development.

Cancers of the Digestive Tract

Adult weight gain significantly increases the risk of oesophageal adenocarcinoma. Excess abdominal fat promotes chronic gastroesophageal reflux disease, which can lead to Barrett's oesophagus, a precancerous condition that may progress to cancer (Spechler, 2013).

Weight gain is also associated with an increased risk of stomach cancer.

Elevated insulin levels associated with obesity increase the risk of pancreatic cancer (Carreras-Torres et al., 2017). In the liver, adult weight gain often leads to non-alcoholic fatty liver disease, disrupting lipid metabolism and increasing the risk of hepatocellular carcinoma (Khan et al., 2015).

Colorectal Cancer

Obesity is strongly linked to colorectal cancer. Increased adiposity elevates circulating insulin and insulin-like growth factor-1 (IGF-1), both of which promote cellular proliferation and inhibit apoptosis, key steps in tumourigenesis (Murphy et al., 2016; Jenab et al., 2007).

Hormone-Related Cancers

In postmenopausal women, adipose tissue becomes the primary source of oestrogen, converting androgens into oestrogens through enzymatic processes. As a result, obese postmenopausal women have higher circulating oestrogen levels.

Elevated insulin further reduces sex hormone–binding globulin, increasing the bioavailability of oestrogen.

These mechanisms explain the increased risk of hormone receptor- positive breast cancer and endometrial cancer observed with adult weight gain (Key et al., 2007; Gunter et al., 2009).

Kidney, Gallbladder, and Reproductive Cancers

Obesity is associated with reduced levels of adiponectin, an insulin-sensitising hormone. Lower adiponectin levels correlate with increased risk of renal cell carcinoma, a risk further amplified by obesity-related hypertension (Liao et al., 2013).

Components of the metabolic syndrome, hyperinsulinemia, hyperglycaemia, dyslipidaemia, and hypertension, intersect with excess body fat and chronic inflammation, increasing the risk of gallbladder cancer.

Adult weight gain is also associated with increased risk of ovarian cancer. In men, obesity is linked to lower testosterone levels, which paradoxically may increase the risk of high-grade prostate cancer (Severi et al., 2006).

Obesity, Immunity, and Viral Persistence

Cervical cancer is caused by persistent infection with human papillomavirus (HPV). Obesity may impair immune function, reducing viral clearance and facilitating progression to malignancy.

Obesity does not cause HPV infection.
It may determine whether the infection resolves, or persists.

The Central Message

Obesity is not a matter of appearance or willpower.
It is a complex biological state that alters hormones, metabolism, inflammation, and immune surveillance.

Adult weight gain, in particular, represents a critical window of preventable risk.

Maintaining a healthy weight is not about achieving an ideal body.
It is about preserving metabolic balance and reducing exposure to biological signals that quietly, persistently promote cancer.

Prevention, once again, lies not in extremes, but in consistency.

Chapter 5

The Cost of Stillness

It was early, but not early enough to feel intentional.

The city was already awake. Screens glowed. Lifts rose and fell. Traffic inched forward in disciplined frustration. Inside an office building, lights flicked on floor by floor. Chairs rolled back. Coffee was poured. Laptops opened. Bodies settled.

No one thought of themselves as inactive.

They had arrived on time. Emails would be answered quickly. Work would be efficient, mentally demanding, productive. Hearts would beat. Lungs would fill. From the outside, everything looked alive.

By midmorning, most of those bodies would still be seated.

Nothing dramatic happened. No pain. No warning. Muscles that once expected to be used remained idle. Glucose lingered longer in the bloodstream than it should. Insulin rose quietly to compensate. Inflammatory signals flickered at low levels, too subtle to feel, but enough to matter. Immune cells patrolled less efficiently.

No single moment stood out as harmful.

By the end of the day, many of these bodies would have spent more than ten hours seated, at desks, in cars, on sofas. No decision would feel reckless. No behaviour would seem extreme.

And yet, taken together, these hours would shape biology more powerfully than many exposures we fear.

Only then do you earn this line:

Cancer does not require catastrophe.
It often requires only time, and conditions that quietly favour it.

What we call *physical inactivity* is not the absence of sport or athleticism. It is the gradual removal of movement from daily life. The replacement of muscle contraction with convenience. The normalisation of stillness as neutral.

It is not neutral.

Physical inactivity rarely announces itself as a problem. It accumulates quietly, an hour seated, a habit formed, a routine hardened. Over time, this stillness alters metabolism, immunity, and risk.

At its core, physical inactivity disrupts energy balance. When energy intake consistently exceeds energy expenditure, the surplus is stored as fat. Movement, of almost any kind, is one of the most effective ways to restore balance.

Physical activity does not have to be athletic to be meaningful. Aerobic activities such as walking, running, or cycling improve cardiovascular fitness, while resistance training strengthens muscle and bone. Recreational movement, household chores, and occupational activity all contribute. What matters most is not perfection, but regularity.

Measuring Movement: The MET Framework

The intensity of physical activity is commonly expressed using the metabolic equivalent of task (MET).
One MET represents the amount of energy expended while sitting quietly at rest.

- **Light-intensity activity** involves less than 3 METs and includes slow walking or standing.
- **Moderate-intensity activity** ranges from 3 to 6 METs and includes brisk walking, cycling at speeds below 16 km/h, or climbing stairs.
- **Vigorous-intensity activity** exceeds 6 METs and includes swimming, tennis, or cycling faster than 16 km/h.

These categories are useful not to label effort, but to help translate movement into biology.

Physical Activity and Cancer Risk

Evidence consistently shows that higher levels of physical activity are associated with lower cancer risk.

One of the largest studies to examine this relationship followed 1.44 million individuals over a median period of 11 years. Participants who engaged in moderate to vigorous physical activity (MET > 3) demonstrated a reduced risk of thirteen different cancers, including cancers of the colon, breast, endometrium, liver, and kidney (Moore et al., 2016).

This relationship follows a dose–response pattern: more movement is generally associated with greater benefit.

An important caveat exists. Increased outdoor physical activity without adequate sun protection may raise the risk of melanoma due to ultraviolet exposure. This risk does not negate the benefits of exercise, it underscores the importance of sensible protection.

Why Movement Protects

Physical activity influences cancer risk through multiple, overlapping mechanisms.

First, it improves insulin sensitivity, reducing circulating insulin levels. Chronic hyperinsulinemia promotes cellular proliferation and inhibits apoptosis, conditions favourable to cancer development.

Second, physical activity reduces chronic inflammation, a central driver of carcinogenesis. Regular movement lowers inflammatory markers and improves immune signalling, shifting the body away from a pro-cancer state.

Third, exercise enhances DNA repair mechanisms, helping cells correct damage before it becomes permanent (Friedenreich et al., 2010).

Fourth, by reducing excess body fat, physical activity lowers circulating oestrogen levels, thereby reducing the risk of hormone receptor–positive breast cancers. Movement also strengthens immune surveillance, improving the body's ability to identify and eliminate abnormal cells.

How Much Is Enough?

Public health recommendations reflect these biological realities.

Adults are advised to engage in:

- At least 150 to 300 minutes of moderate-intensity physical activity per week, or
- 75 to 100 minutes of vigorous-intensity activity per week,
  or a combination of both.

These are not performance goals. They are thresholds at which biological benefit becomes reliable.

The Gap Between Knowledge and Action

Despite clear evidence, many populations fall short of these recommendations.

Surveys indicate that only 64% of men and 60% of women in England meet minimum physical activity guidelines. Rates are lower in Wales and Ireland, and only modestly higher in Scotland (Sport England, 2016; National Survey, 2016; Scottish Survey, 2017; Health Survey, 2017).

This gap is not a failure of motivation, it is a failure of environment, routine, and priority.

Movement as Prevention

Physical activity is not a treatment for cancer. It is something quieter and more powerful: a form of prevention woven into daily life.

Movement recalibrates metabolism, tempers inflammation, strengthens immunity, and restores balance. It does not require special equipment or extreme discipline. It requires consistency.

In a world designed for stillness, choosing to move is not optional biology, it is protective biology.

Chapter 6

Washoku: A Sustainable Anti-Cancer Diet for a Sustainable Planet

The first thing I noticed was the silence.

It was early evening in Japan, the hour when kitchens are active but restrained. There was no clatter, no urgency. I was seated at a small wooden table, watching a meal arrive in pieces rather than as a single declaration.

A bowl of miso soup.
Steamed rice.
Grilled fish no larger than my palm.
Pickled vegetables arranged with care.

Nothing extravagant.
Nothing excessive.

No one spoke about calories.
No one spoke about antioxidants.
No one spoke about cancer.

Yet everything on the table was doing biological work.

The food followed the season. Portions respected appetite rather than indulgence. There was protein, but it did not dominate the plate. Vegetables were not decoration; they were structure. Fermentation was not a trend, but tradition.

Even the pace of eating felt deliberate, as if the body were being given time to listen to itself.

What struck me most was not what was present, but what was absent.

There was no sense of restriction.
No moral language around food.
No performance of health.

Just quiet consistency, repeated daily across decades.

Only later did I learn the word for this way of eating: Washoku. Literally, it means Japanese food. But the deeper meaning is harmony, between food and season, nourishment and restraint, human biology and the natural world.

The more I studied cancer biology, the more that meal returned to me, not as nostalgia, but as data.

Japan, among developed nations, consistently demonstrates exceptional longevity. That meal did not explain the statistic on its own. But it made the question unavoidable:

What if cancer prevention is not hidden in dramatic interventions, but embedded in ordinary patterns repeated over a lifetime?

Alcohol, tobacco, and unsafe sexual practices are well-established contributors to premature mortality. Yet another risk factor, often underestimated because it is normalised, may rival them in long-term impact: an unhealthy diet.

As the global population approaches ten billion by 2050, the challenge of providing a diet that is both cancer-protective and environmentally sustainable becomes daunting. While global food systems require policy-level solutions, individual understanding remains critical. Knowing *what* to eat, and *why*, is one of the few preventive tools available to everyone.

Modern diets are dominated by processed and ultra-processed foods. Even home-cooked meals frequently centre on red meat or poultry accompanied by refined starches such as potatoes or white rice, meals dense in calories but poor in fibre, phytochemicals, and microbial substrates. Over time, this dietary pattern fuels obesity, inflammation, metabolic dysfunction, and cancer risk.

The phrase *"you are what you eat"* is not a metaphor. It is a biological reality.

6.1 Washoku: Dietary Harmony as Biology

Among developed nations, Japan consistently demonstrates exceptional longevity. A key contributor may be Washoku, the traditional Japanese dietary pattern. The term itself conveys harmony, between food and season, nourishment and restraint, humans and nature.

Washoku emphasises:

- seasonal ingredients,
- high intake of seafood, soy, vegetables, and green tea,
- low consumption of red meat and refined sugars.

Large population studies associate this pattern with reduced cancer risk and improved longevity (Yatsuya et al., 2021).

Importantly, Washoku is not unique. Many traditional cultures, including South Indian dietary practices such as eating from banana leaves, once followed food systems closely aligned with nature. These systems were gradually displaced by industrialised, highly processed foods that maximise convenience at the expense of biology.

6.2 Whole Foods Over Supplements

An effective anti-cancer diet must be fibre-rich ($\geq$30 g/day), plant-forward, and minimally processed. Daily intake of fruits and non-starchy vegetables should exceed 400g to derive measurable long-term benefit.

Crucially, the benefits described in this chapter arise from whole foods, not supplements. Isolated compounds often fail to replicate the synergistic effects of foods consumed in their natural matrix. Moreover, supplement studies are limited by uncertain composition and lack of commercial incentive for rigorous testing.

Food is not chemistry alone.
It is context.

6.3 Foods That Protect Through the Gut Microbiome

The gut microbiome is central to dietary cancer prevention. Many bioactive compounds require microbial transformation to exert their effects.

Apples

Apples contain triterpenoids, flavanols, and fibre, which reduce the risk of lung and oestrogen-receptor-negative breast cancers. Fermentable apple fibres are metabolised by gut bacteria into short-chain fatty acids such as butyrate, which protect against colorectal cancer and suppress inflammation.

Blueberries (Star Candidate)

Blueberries are rich in vitamin C, flavanols, phenolic acids, anthocyanins, tannins, stilbenes, and other antioxidants. Of particular importance are ellagitannins, which are converted by gut microbes into ellagic acid and subsequently into urolithins, compounds that reduce DNA damage and exert anti-inflammatory and anti-proliferative effects.

Importantly, the benefit derived from blueberries varies between individuals, depending on microbiome composition (Inhae Kang et al., 2016).

Raspberries (Star Candidate)

Raspberries contain ellagitannins, phenolic acids, vitamin C, anthocyanins, and fibre. Black raspberries enhance tumour immunosurveillance, preventing malignant cells from establishing dominance (Pan et al., 2017). They have also been shown to prevent progression of Barrett's oesophagus to oesophageal cancer (Kresty et al., 2016), reduce oral cancer risk (Oghumu et al., 2017), and modulate the gut microbiome to protect against colorectal cancer (Peiffer et al., 2020).

Cranberries (Star Candidate)

Cranberries contain terpenes, proanthocyanidins, tannins, phenolic acids, flavanols, and anthocyanins. Unique cranberry proanthocyanidins inhibit proliferation and induce apoptosis in multiple cancer models, including glioblastoma (Ferguson et al., 2006), lymphoma (Hochman et al., 2008), prostate, colon, oesophageal, lung, gastric, ovarian (Deziel et al., 2010), and bladder cancers (Prasain et al., 2008).

6.4 Fruits That Modulate Hormonal and Oxidative Pathways

Grapes (the fruit, not wine)

Grapes contain resveratrol, phenolic acids, proanthocyanidins, ellagitannins, flavanols, anthocyanins, and tannins, concentrated in the skin and seeds. Resveratrol acts as a phytoestrogen, competing with endogenous oestrogens at receptor sites, potentially reducing the risk of hormone-positive breast cancer. Over 570 PubMed-indexed studies have explored this interaction.

Consumption of 1.1–1.8 servings of grapes daily has been associated with reduced skin cancer risk (Singh et al., 2017).

Oranges and Citrus Fruits

Citrus fruits provide naringenin, flavanones, terpenes, dietary fibre, and vitamin C. Citrus intake is associated with reduced lung cancer risk (Wang et al., 2021) and suggestive protection against gastric cancer (Bertuccio et al., 2019).

Nobiletin, derived from citrus peel, inhibits aberrant cell proliferation and induces death of mutant cells, though limited bioavailability and pesticide exposure complicate its practical use (Goh et al., 2019).

Strawberries (Star Candidate)

Strawberries contain stilbenes, vitamin C, flavan-3-ols, fibre, ellagitannins, proanthocyanidins, and anthocyanins. Higher intake is associated with reduced risk of hormone-negative breast cancer (Jung et al., 2013). The Romina variety has demonstrated particular efficacy against ovarian cancer models (Haq et al., 2020).

6.5 Vegetables as cellular defense systems

Tomatoes

Tomatoes contain lycopene, phytoene, phytofluene, β-carotene, and vitamin C. Lycopene accumulates in the skin, offering protection against UV-induced damage. Whole tomatoes outperform lycopene supplements, with tangerine tomatoes showing superior bioavailability (Cooperstone et al., 2017). Tomato glycoalkaloids such as tomatidine further contribute to photoprotection and cancer prevention.

Cruciferous Vegetables (Broccoli as a model)

Cruciferous vegetables contain sulforaphane, produced from glucoraphanin through enzymatic reactions involving myrosinase, a process completed in part by the gut microbiome.

Sulforaphane activates Nrf2, a master regulator of cellular defense against oxidative stress and inflammation. It also inhibits histone deacetylases, linking diet directly to epigenetic regulation of cancer (Laura et al., 2018).

Sulforaphane demonstrates activity against antibiotic-resistant *Helicobacter pylori* and reduces gastric cancer risk (Fahey et al., 2002). Physical activity appears to enhance sulforaphane's bioactivity, reinforcing the interdependence of diet and lifestyle.

Carrots

Carrots provide phenolic acids, falcarinol, and carotenoids. Consumption of ≥32 g per day was associated with a 17% reduction in colorectal cancer risk in a Danish cohort (Deding et al., 2020). A meta-analysis reported a 42% reduction in lung cancer risk (Xu et al., 2019). β-carotene supplementation, particularly in smokers, is contraindicated, highlighting the importance of whole-food context.

Spinach

Spinach contains β-carotene, lutein, zeaxanthin, folate, vitamin K, fibre, flavanols, and bioactive lipids such as monogalactosyldiacylglycerol, which inhibits breast and colon cancer cell proliferation (Abedin et al., 2021; Fornaciari et al., 2015). Spinach also supports a healthy gut microbiome (Zheng et al., 2021).

6.6 Foods with Longstanding Cultural and Biological Evidence

Garlic

Garlic contains organosulfur compounds, saponins, polysaccharides, and phenolics. Historically used across civilisations, garlic demonstrates antimicrobial activity against *Helicobacter pylori* and reduces gastric cancer risk (Li et al., 2019). Case-control studies associate garlic consumption with reduced colorectal, lung, oral, renal, ovarian, and oesophageal cancer risk.

Soy

Soy provides genistein, daidzein, glycitein, fibre, lignans, and folate. Data from the China Kadoorie Biobank indicate reduced breast cancer risk with higher soy intake (Wei et al., 2020). Genistein inhibits *H. pylori* and suppresses NF-κB–mediated inflammation, contributing to protection against gastric and bladder cancers (Merga et al., 2016; Wada et al., 2018).

Turmeric (Star Candidate)

Turmeric contains curcumin, a polyphenol with pleiotropic anti-cancer effects. Curcumin inhibits epidermal growth factor receptor signalling (Tikhomirov et al., 2003), enhances apoptosis (Watson et al., 2010), suppresses NF-κB, and demonstrates efficacy against multiple cancer cell lines including triple-negative breast cancer and colorectal cancer (Pignanelli et al., 2017).

6.7 Whole Grains, Nuts, and Protective Beverages

Whole Grains

Whole grains retain the bran, germ, and endosperm, providing fibre, antioxidants, phenolic acids, lignans, and minerals. Consumption is associated with reduced colorectal (Aune et al., 2011) and breast cancer risk

(McKenzie et al., 2015). Denmark's Whole Grain Partnership illustrates how population-level dietary change is achievable.

Walnuts

Walnuts contain omega-3 fatty acids, ellagitannins, melatonin, and polyphenols, modulating inflammation, immunity, and the microbiome. Walnut intake is associated with reduced colorectal, breast, and oesophageal cancer risk (Chen et al., 2019).

Coffee and Green Tea

Coffee provides chlorogenic acids, cafestol, kahweol, lignans, and melanoidins. UK Biobank data associate coffee consumption with reduced hepatocellular carcinoma risk (Tran et al., 2019). Green tea polyphenols such as epigallocatechin-3-gallate reduce endometrial and prostate cancer risk in dose-dependent manners.

A Closing Synthesis

An anti-cancer diet is not a checklist.
It is a pattern, plant-forward, fibre-rich, minimally processed, microbiome-supportive, and seasonally grounded.

Washoku is one expression of this principle, but the biology is universal. Such a diet protects human health while demanding less from the planet, a rare convergence of personal and planetary benefit.

Food is not merely fuel.
It is instruction.

And over decades, those instructions shape destiny.

Chapter 7

Tobacco: A Gift to Columbus and the Longest Pandemic in History

The leaves were passed from hand to hand without ceremony.

They were dry, brittle at the edges, wrapped loosely in woven fibre. The air was heavy with salt and heat as the small boat rocked gently against the shore of Guanahani. The men who offered the leaves did so as they offered fruit, water, and gestures of welcome, with curiosity, not calculation.

Christopher Columbus examined them briefly.

He did not ask what they were for. He did not ask why they mattered. Unfamiliar and unremarkable, the leaves held no obvious value. Accounts suggest he discarded them, perhaps into the sea, as casually as one sheds ballast. His own gifts in return, hats and trinkets, were no better understood.

The exchange passed without comment.

No one present could have known that this moment, unremarkable, asymmetrical, unrecorded in any official log, would mark the beginning of a global catastrophe. There was no smoke yet. No cough. No craving. No tumour growing invisibly decades later.

Just leaves, sunlight, and the quiet confidence of assuming that what one does not understand cannot matter.

The Indigenous peoples who cultivated tobacco used it sparingly. It was bound to ritual, illness, and meaning. Its power was contained by context. What crossed the ocean was not merely a plant, but its removal from restraint.

Pandemics do not always announce themselves.

Some arrive without urgency.
Some require centuries.
Some are carried not by droplets, but by commerce.

Long before COVID-19, humanity was already living through a pandemic, one that spread slowly, silently, and deliberately.

Tobacco.

Only now does the explanation begin.

7.1 How Tobacco Left the Americas

Tobacco belongs to the same botanical family as nightshades, peppers, and potatoes. Indigenous populations of the Americas, including Native Americans and the

Mayans, used tobacco as early as 1000 BC, primarily in religious rituals and medicinal contexts. Its use was controlled, ceremonial, and limited.

That restraint would not survive colonisation.

In 1492, Christopher Columbus docked at a Caribbean island known to its inhabitants as Guanahani. Unaware that Columbus had renamed their home San Salvador and claimed it for the Spanish monarchy, the islanders welcomed him and offered gifts, including dried tobacco leaves.

Columbus, unfamiliar with their use, reportedly discarded the leaves. On subsequent voyages, particularly in present-day Cuba, he encountered tobacco again. This time, curiosity replaced indifference.

Tobacco crossed the Atlantic.

Its widespread adoption, however, is most closely associated with Jean Nicot de Villemain, a French diplomat appointed ambassador to Lisbon by King Henry II. Convinced that tobacco possessed medicinal properties, Nicot sent tobacco leaves and powdered snuff to Paris in 1560, encouraging the Queen to inhale it as a remedy for headaches.

The practice spread rapidly. By the seventeenth century, tobacco, especially in powdered form as snuff, had become fashionable across Europe, particularly in the United Kingdom.

7.2 Early Warnings Ignored

King James I of England was among the first to tax tobacco, and later, among the first to recognise its dangers. He condemned tobacco use publicly and attempted regulation, supported at times by the Church.

It did not matter.

By the eighteenth century, tobacco cultivation had expanded globally. The plant was formally named *Nicotiana* by the Swedish naturalist Carolus Linnaeus, after Jean Nicot. Its active compound was later identified and named nicotine.

Neither Nicot nor the Indigenous peoples who first used tobacco could have imagined the scale of harm to come.

7.3 Tobacco as a Modern Carcinogen

Today, tobacco is responsible for approximately 7.3 million deaths each year worldwide. Each individual who dies from tobacco-related disease loses, on average, 15 years of active life, often during middle age, when professional, familial, and social responsibilities are greatest.

If current trends continue, tobacco will cause over one billion premature deaths in this century alone.

What makes tobacco unique among carcinogens is not only its lethality, but its protection.

7.4 The Tobacco Industry and Manufactured Doubt

By the early 1960s, tobacco manufacturers understood nicotine far better than the public, or governments, did.

Internal research projects such as Project Hippo I and Hippo II, conducted at the Battelle Memorial Institute in Geneva, examined nicotine's pharmacology and toxicity. The findings were unambiguous: nicotine was addictive and harmful.

This information was withheld.

The purpose of tobacco research was never consumer safety. It was optimisation of dependence.

Manufacturers introduced filters, claiming reduced harm. In reality, filters diluted smoke with air, making inhalation smoother and deeper. In 2014, the US Surgeon General confirmed the consequence: a rise in lung adenocarcinoma following the widespread adoption of filtered cigarettes, as carcinogens were driven deeper into peripheral lung tissue (Song et al., 2017).

The deception did not end there.

Ammonia was added to tobacco blends, altering nicotine's pH and dramatically increasing its ability to cross the blood–brain barrier. Each inhalation delivered nicotine faster and more efficiently, reinforcing addiction with every puff.

This was not ignorance.

It was engineering.

7.5 Tobacco and Cancer

Smoking is causally linked to at least fourteen cancers, including cancers of the lung, pancreas, bladder, bowel, kidney, stomach, oesophagus, larynx, liver, ovaries, cervix, mouth, and upper throat.

Definitive proof came not from industry, but from independent science.

British physician Richard Doll and epidemiologist Austin Bradford Hill first demonstrated the link between smoking and lung cancer. Facing fierce resistance, they pursued stronger evidence.

That evidence emerged through the British Doctors Study, conducted by Doll and Richard Peto, which followed tens of thousands of physicians in the United Kingdom for over half a century.

- The 40-year follow-up confirmed dramatic increases in cancer mortality among smokers (Doll et al., 1994).
- The 50-year follow-up demonstrated that smokers lose nearly 10 years of healthy life, with increased mortality from multiple cancers and cardiovascular disease (Doll et al., 2004).

7.6 The Power of Cessation

The most important finding of the British Doctors Study was not about death, but about reversibility.

- Smoking cessation at 30 years of age reduced cancer risk almost to that of never-smokers.
- Cessation at 50 years of age halved the risk of cancer-related death.

In other words: quitting works.

Risk does not vanish overnight, but the body begins repairing itself almost immediately. The longer one remains smoke-free, the greater the benefit.

A Preventable Tragedy

Tobacco is not a lifestyle choice in the conventional sense. It is a commercially sustained addiction, engineered for dependence and protected by decades of misinformation.

No anti-cancer strategy is complete without confronting tobacco directly.

The recommendation is unequivocal:

- Avoid smoking.
- Avoid passive smoking.
- If you smoke, stop, at any age.

This is not moral advice.

It is biological fact.

Tobacco is the longest-running pandemic in human history, and unlike most pandemics, its cure is already known.

Chapter 8

Alcohol: A Toast to Cancer

The glasses were already raised.

It was a small gathering, the kind that feels harmless by design. A birthday. A promotion. Someone had brought a bottle they'd been saving, its label handled with the care usually reserved for photographs or heirlooms. The cork came out cleanly. The liquid caught the light.

There was laughter. A pause. The practiced choreography of pouring, clinking, sipping.

No one mentioned cancer.
No one ever does.

The first sip burned briefly, then softened. Faces relaxed. Conversation loosened. The moment did what moments like this are meant to do: it felt safe.

What happened next was invisible.

Within minutes, the alcohol left the glass and entered the bloodstream. No sensation marked the change. No warning accompanied it. A molecule encountered an enzyme. A reaction occurred.

A new compound formed.

There was no pain when it appeared.
No alarm when it bound to DNA.
No awareness when repair mechanisms faltered, or when immune vigilance dimmed.

The celebration continued.

Biology, meanwhile, took notes.

Nearly three decades ago, the World Health Organisation classified alcohol as a **Group 1 carcinogen**. What makes this designation unsettling is not only its scientific certainty, but its cultural invisibility.

Alcohol is rarely perceived as a carcinogen. It is celebrated, ritualised, and normalised. Yet its primary metabolic by-product, **acetaldehyde**, is among the most potent carcinogens encountered in daily life.

8.1 From Fermentation to DNA Damage

Ethanol (alcohol) is produced through microbial fermentation:

- from grains and starches,
- and from fruit carbohydrates via yeast metabolism.

Upon consumption, ethanol is converted in the body to acetaldehyde by the enzyme alcohol dehydrogenase.

Acetaldehyde is not a benign intermediate. It is a highly reactive molecule with profound biological consequences.

It interferes with DNA repair by inhibiting enzymes required to correct damaged DNA. It reduces folate absorption, depriving cells of a key substrate for DNA synthesis and repair. It lowers retinoic acid levels, a compound involved in cellular differentiation and cancer prevention.

At the chromosomal level, acetaldehyde induces:

- DNA adduct formation,
- strand breaks,
- chromosomal aberrations,
- and altered DNA methylation, an epigenetic change that can silence tumour suppressor genes.

Together, these effects increase the probability that damaged cells survive, replicate, and evolve into malignancy (Seitz et al., 2010).

8.2 Genetic Vulnerability Does Not Equal Safety

Under normal circumstances, acetaldehyde is converted to acetate, a harmless molecule that cells can use as an energy source, by the enzyme acetaldehyde dehydrogenase (ALDH).

However, ALDH exists in multiple isoforms, and genetic variations can significantly reduce its activity. Deficient ALDH function leads to accumulation of acetaldehyde after alcohol consumption.

This deficiency is particularly common among individuals of East Asian ancestry, including Japanese and Chinese populations, and manifests clinically as facial flushing after alcohol intake.

Importantly, genetic protection is relative, not absolute. Even in individuals with fully functional ALDH, acetaldehyde levels rise with each drink. Cancer risk increases incrementally, there is no safe threshold.

8.3 Alcohol-Associated Cancers

Alcohol consumption is causally linked to cancers of the:

- oesophagus,
- breast,
- colorectum,
- liver,
- larynx,
- and pharynx.

Among women, alcohol increases circulating oestrogen levels, contributing to an elevated risk of hormone receptor–positive breast cancer.

Alcohol also acts synergistically with tobacco. Individuals who both smoke and drink are not exposed to additive risk, but to multiplicative risk, a biological collaboration between two carcinogens.

8.4 Alcohol and Immune Suppression

Cancer prevention relies heavily on immune surveillance. The immune system continuously identifies and eliminates cells undergoing malignant transformation.

Alcohol disrupts this process.

Experimental studies demonstrate that alcohol consumption impairs antitumour immunity, particularly by reducing the activity of cytotoxic $CD8^+$ T cells, which are central to recognising and destroying cancerous cells (Meadows et al., 2015).

This immune suppression does not require heavy drinking. It is dose-dependent and cumulative.

8.5 "Just One Drink": A Misleading Comfort

The argument for moderation often rests on familiarity: *one drink per day can't matter*. To understand why this belief is flawed, it is instructive to examine a less emotional exposure pathway.

Several studies have investigated alcohol-based mouthwashes.

The Alcohol-Related Cancers and Genetic Susceptibility in Europe (ARCAGE) study demonstrated a significant increase in cancer risk among individuals who used alcohol-based mouthwash three times daily (Ahrens et al., 2014).

The INHANCE study further showed that using alcohol-based mouthwash more than once per day for 35 years increased the risk of oral cancer (Boffetta et al., 2016).

These findings are difficult to dismiss because they remove intoxication, social context, and lifestyle confounders. They isolate acetaldehyde exposure, and reveal its carcinogenic potential even at localised, repeated doses.

8.6 Awareness Without Alarm

Not everyone who drinks alcohol will develop cancer. Risk is probabilistic, not deterministic.

But population-level risk matters.

Alcohol is not an elixir of longevity. It is better understood as a dose-dependent carcinogen, normalised by culture and underestimated by perception.

Awareness alone can change behaviour. Keeping a diary or using an application to track alcohol intake helps restore visibility to an otherwise invisible risk. Reduction, rather than absolutism, is often the most sustainable first step.

A Measured Conclusion

Alcohol does not confer protection against cancer.
It compromises DNA repair, alters epigenetic regulation, disrupts immune surveillance, and increases hormonal signalling that favours tumour development.

The most effective cancer-preventive strategy with respect to alcohol is simple:
less is better, and none is best.

This is not a call for abstinence.
It is a call for clarity.

A toast, once in a while, may mark celebration.
But biology remembers every exposure.

Chapter 9

The Mind as Terrain: Psychological Stress and Cancer Risk

She sat across from me without crying.

That was what struck me first.

Her posture was composed, almost formal, hands folded neatly in her lap. She spoke clearly, methodically, as if recounting a schedule rather than a life. In a matter of minutes, she mentioned the death of her husband, the loss of her job, a prolonged legal dispute with her family, and the responsibility of caring for an elderly parent.

Each event was delivered with the same even cadence.

"I'm managing," she said, anticipating the question before I asked it.

Her blood pressure was elevated. Her sleep was fragmented. She had lost weight unintentionally. Her immune markers, though still within reference ranges, had begun to drift. None of this surprised her. Strain, she explained, had become permanent.

What concerned me was not any single symptom.

It was the absence of recovery.

There was no pause.
No return to baseline.
No moment when the body was allowed to stand down.

Long after the appointment ended, I found myself thinking about how often composure is mistaken for resilience, and how easily unexpressed distress becomes invisible, not only to others, but eventually to the person carrying it.

The body does not interpret endurance as strength.
It interprets it as threat.

In medicine, we are trained to look for causes that can be isolated, targeted, and removed. Psychological stress resists that instinct. It leaves no lesion, no pathogen, no single mutation. Yet it moves relentlessly through physiology, shaping immune responses, inflammatory tone, and cellular repair.

The question is not whether stress causes cancer.

The question is whether it alters the biological landscape in which disease must either be restrained, or allowed to advance.

As we grow older, many of us forget a simple truth: the purpose of life is not endurance, but experience. Loss, injustice, and failure are inevitable. How these experiences are carried within the mind may matter more than the events themselves.

The mind is not separate from the body.
It is embedded within it.

Modern biology increasingly recognises that psychological states are translated into biochemical signals, signals that shape immunity, inflammation, metabolism, and cellular repair. The mind does not cause cancer. But it may influence the terrain in which cancer arises.

9.1 What Stress Does to the Body

Stress is not merely a mental event. It is a whole-body response.

When faced with danger, physical or perceived, the body activates the sympathetic nervous system and the hypothalamic–pituitary–adrenal (HPA) axis. Stress hormones such as adrenaline and cortisol surge. Heart rate accelerates. Blood pressure rises. Glucose floods the bloodstream. Blood flow is redirected toward the brain, heart, and skeletal muscle.

These responses are adaptive when threats are brief.

The problem arises when stress does not resolve.

In modern life, threats rarely end cleanly. Prolonged grief, financial insecurity, caregiving burden, racism, interpersonal conflict, and sustained uncertainty can keep stress pathways continuously activated. Chronic stress has been shown to:

- impair immune surveillance,
- promote low-grade inflammation,
- disrupt DNA repair mechanisms,
- and accelerate telomere shortening.

These changes do not create cancer.
They reduce the body's ability to prevent it.

9.2 Historical observations: Before molecular biology

Long before molecular pathways were understood, physicians noticed patterns.

Galen, personal physician to Emperor Marcus Aurelius, observed that women who were persistently melancholic appeared more prone to cancer than those who were emotionally content. These were not claims of causation, but clinical impressions, attempts to name vulnerability before mechanisms existed.

In 1402, Maestro Lorenzo Sassoli warned:

"What displeases me is your being grieved and taking all matters to heart…
for it is this, as the whole of physic teaches, which destroys our body more than any other cause."

By the 19th century, such ideas were no longer fringe.

Walter Hayle Walshe proposed that inherited susceptibility might be exacerbated by psychological strain. Sir James Paget observed that profound anxiety and deferred hope often preceded cancer progression.

They were not assigning blame.
They were describing patterns.

9.3 Early attempts to systematise the mind-cancer link

In 1802, the Society for the Prevention and Cure of Cancer included among its core research questions:

"Is there a predisposing temperament?"
(Hoffman, 1915)

Later observers attempted to formalise this idea, sometimes too eagerly.

Herbert Lumley Snow reported that many patients with breast and uterine cancer experienced profound emotional distress prior to diagnosis (Snow, 1893). Peller observed higher cancer mortality among widowed women compared with unmarried women, even after accounting for known confounders (Peller, 1940).

These studies were limited by methodology and bias. They cannot be interpreted as proof. But they consistently pointed toward psychological vulnerability as a modifier of disease course, not its origin.

9.4 When speculation went too far

Some historical interpretations overreached.

Franz Anton Mesmer's concept of "animal magnetism" and later hypnosis attempted to explain disease through invisible forces. Byron Butler proposed a distinct "cancer personality," describing individuals with suppressed anger or excessive self-sacrifice (Butler, 1954). Orbach even suggested intergenerational emotional disturbance in mothers of children with leukaemia (Orbach, 1955).

These ideas lack scientific rigor and are no longer accepted. They remind us of the danger of blaming patients for their illness, a mistake modern medicine must avoid at all costs.

Stress does not cause cancer.
No personality produces tumours.

9.5 Modern Biology: Where the Evidence Now Stands

What contemporary research does support is more precise, and more cautious.

Chronic psychological stress can:

- suppress cytotoxic immune responses,
- increase pro-inflammatory signalling,
- impair DNA repair capacity,
- and accelerate biological aging.

These changes may influence cancer progression, recurrence, and outcomes, particularly in individuals with existing genetic or environmental risk factors.

The relationship is probabilistic, not deterministic.

9.6 A Humane Conclusion

Carrying unrelenting psychological burden alters biology.

Peace of mind does not guarantee health.
But persistent despair can erode resilience.

Relying on a single emotional anchor makes one vulnerable to collapse if that support is lost. Sharing distress, seeking help, cultivating multiple sources of meaning, these are not philosophical luxuries. They are biological strategies.

Quality of life may not determine destiny.
But it shapes the terrain on which destiny unfolds.

And over time, that terrain matters.

A Pause

Up to this point, this book has asked you to look at cancer from a distance.

At patterns.
At populations.
At habits that quietly accumulate over years.

Diet.
Sleep.
Movement.
Light.
Stress.
Toxins.

These forces shape risk long before disease announces itself. They work slowly, invisibly, often unnoticed. When prevention succeeds, nothing happens, and that silence is easy to dismiss.

But cancer does not arise only from general risk. It also follows specific pathways, exploits known vulnerabilities, and depends on timing.

Some cancers wait for a virus.
Some wait for chronic inflammation.
Some wait for a missed screening.
Some wait for years, until prevention arrives too late.

The chapters that follow move closer still. They are not about averages, but about interception. Not about what might help, but about what does, for the right person, at the right time.

This is where prevention becomes precise.

Not everyone needs the same intervention.
But everyone deserves to know which ones matter to them.

What follows is not a list of instructions, but a map, drawn from evidence, experience, and consequence.

You may not need every path described ahead.
But knowing where they lead may change how, and when, you choose to act.

Precision Prevention

Right Intervention. Right Time. Right Individual.

Some cancers can be intercepted.

Not with fear.
Not with guesswork.
But with timing, biology, and evidence.

What follows is about acting early, and acting precisely, when it matters most.

Chapter 9½

Aging, Mutations, and Time: The Silent Platform

There are moments when nothing appears to happen.

The train has not arrived.
No gate has closed.
The platform looks exactly as it did a moment ago.

And yet, something irreversible has already occurred.

At King's Cross Station, between Platforms 9 and 10, there is a place most people pass without noticing. No sign announces it. No alarm sounds. But once crossed, you are no longer where you were before.

Time works much the same way in biology.

We do not feel the crossing.
We only realise, later, that the rules have changed.

Cancer does not arrive suddenly.
It appears after the passage has already been made.

Time as the Unseen Exposure

Every cell carries a record.

With each division, DNA is copied.
With each repair, a correction is attempted.
With every inflammatory signal, metabolic fluctuation, or
environmental insult, small changes are introduced.

Most are fixed.
Some are tolerated.
A few persist.

From birth, we move forward one division at a time.

By adolescence, billions of replications have occurred.
By midlife, trillions.
By later decades, the cumulative burden becomes
biologically meaningful.

Aging is not a disease.

It is the most powerful exposure we will ever experience.

Not because it guarantees cancer,
but because it makes everything else matter more.

Crossing the Threshold

For years, the body compensates.

Surveillance systems detect errors.
Immune cells intervene.
Tissue architecture is preserved.

We feel well.
We function normally.
Nothing appears wrong.

Then, quietly, a threshold is crossed.

A cell acquires a mutation that confers advantage.
Another follows.
A small population expands.
Architecture subtly shifts.

These changes do not announce themselves with pain or dysfunction. They coexist easily with health.

One of the clearest examples is clonal haematopoiesis of indeterminate potential (CHIP), the age-associated expansion of blood cell clones carrying mutations commonly seen in cancer.

Most individuals with CHIP will never develop leukaemia.

But its existence reveals something essential:

Precancerous states are common.
What is rare is noticing when we pass them.

Cancer, in most cases, is not the first event.
It is the last.

Why Screening Exists

Screening is often misunderstood, as intrusion, as alarmism, as something to postpone.

In truth, screening is an acknowledgment that time has direction.

Cancers such as breast, colorectal, and cervical cancer do not arise overnight. They progress through identifiable, interruptible stages. Screening works because biology moves slowly, until it doesn't.

Screening schedules are not arbitrary.
They are mapped to mutation rates, growth kinetics, and windows of reversibility.

To ignore screening is not to remain safely on the platform.

It is simply to cross without looking.

Delay does not stop cancer.
It allows time to finish its work.

Why Prevention Matters More After Midlife

There is a comforting myth that prevention belongs to youth.

Biology disagrees.

As mutations accumulate, marginal risks gain leverage:

- chronic inflammation,
- metabolic dysfunction,
- immune fatigue,
- circadian disruption,
- cumulative toxin exposure.

These factors rarely initiate cancer on their own.

They accelerate trajectories already in motion.

After midlife, prevention is no longer about eliminating risk.
It is about slowing progression, restoring balance, and supporting surveillance systems that, remarkably, still function when given the chance.

Once the crossing has occurred,
small advantages matter more.

Aging is not destiny

Time cannot be reversed.

Its consequences, however, are not fixed.

Populations that maintain physical activity, metabolic health, immune competence, restorative sleep, and adherence to screening do not escape cancer entirely, but they delay it, soften its course, and improve survival.

Aging increases vulnerability.
Lifestyle determines how that vulnerability is expressed.

From Here On

This chapter sits where it does for a reason.

Until now, we have focused on shared foundations, diet, movement, sleep, environment, mental well-being. These remain essential.

Beyond this point, prevention becomes increasingly individual.

Genetics.
Family history.
Prior exposures.
Timing.

This is where precision prevention begins, not as a replacement for earlier strategies, but as their natural continuation.

We have crossed the platform.
Time has already moved us forward.

What we do next still matters.

Chapter 10

Precision Prevention of Breast Cancer

The waiting room was quieter than expected.

Not silent, just subdued, in the way hospital spaces become when everyone inside is doing mental arithmetic they have not yet learned how to say out loud. A woman in her thirties sat across from me, scrolling absently on her phone, pausing every few seconds as if she had forgotten why she was holding it. Her coat was still on.

People keep their coats on when they believe they will not be there long.

She had not come because she felt unwell.
She had come because a screening image, taken routinely, almost casually, had asked a question.

There were no symptoms. No pain. No warning signs she could point to in retrospect. Just a letter, a follow-up appointment, and now this room.

When her name was called, she stood quickly, smoothing her sleeve in a reflexive gesture that suggested control where little existed. The door closed behind her with a soft click. The rest of us waited.

Breast cancer often enters lives like this, not with drama, but with interruption. It intrudes on normalcy. It reframes age, plans, and assumptions about time. And when it appears early, in women who do not fit the expected profile, it leaves a particular kind of disbelief in its wake.

This is the moment most people imagine when they think of breast cancer.

But the biology began long before the letter arrived.

Precision prevention begins there, long before the waiting room.

Globally, breast cancer is one of the most diagnosed cancers and remains the leading cause of cancer among women. Approximately one in twenty women will be diagnosed during their lifetime, with even higher incidence in high-income countries. While the majority of cases occur after menopause, nearly 7% are diagnosed in women under the age of 40 (Cancer Research UK).

That distribution matters.

It tells us that breast cancer is not governed by age alone, nor by chance in isolation. It reflects a long biological conversation, between hormones, development, reproduction, genetics, and time, that begins decades before a tumour is ever visible.

Beyond the lifestyle factors discussed earlier in this book, several reproductive, hormonal, genetic, and screening-related variables significantly influence breast cancer risk.

Understanding them allows prevention to become precise rather than generic.

10.1 Age at Menarche

The age of onset of menstruation (menarche) has declined globally over recent decades. Earlier menarche increases cumulative lifetime exposure to oestrogen and progesterone.

Epidemiological data indicate that breast cancer risk increases by approximately 5% for each year earlier at menarche compared with peers within the same population (Sisti et al., 2016).

Factors associated with earlier menarche include:

- cigarette smoking,
- chronic psychological stress,
- excessive sugar intake,
- and weight gain during pregnancy, which may influence the age of menarche in daughters (Boynton et al., 2011).

While menarche timing is not fully modifiable, these associations underscore the intergenerational impact of metabolic and environmental health.

10.2 Childbearing and Breast Cancer Risk

Some of the earliest insights into reproductive influences on breast cancer came from observations among nuns, who exhibited higher rates of breast cancer due to lifelong nulliparity.

Childbearing reduces the risk of oestrogen receptor–positive breast cancer, but only when it occurs before a certain age.

Key findings include:

- Childbearing before 35 years of age is associated with reduced breast cancer risk.
- Childbearing after 35 years of age is associated with a *transient increase* in risk compared with nulliparous women.
- Very early first childbirth (before age 20) is associated with up to a 70% reduction in lifetime breast cancer risk (MacMahon et al., 1970; Albrektsen et al., 2005).

Importantly, childbirth is associated with a short-term increase in breast cancer risk in the years immediately following delivery, followed by a long-term protective effect that becomes evident approximately 10 years postpartum (Lambe et al., 1994).

Proposed mechanisms include:

- reduced sensitivity of breast tissue to oestrogen,
- a decrease in the number of vulnerable mammary stem cells,
- and immune-mediated remodelling during the postpartum period.

These observations are biological, not prescriptive. Decisions about childbearing are deeply personal and shaped by social, economic, health, and ethical considerations. Precision prevention does not mandate choices, it clarifies consequences, allowing informed autonomy.

10.3 Breastfeeding

Breastfeeding confers additional protection.

For every 12 months of cumulative breastfeeding, breast cancer risk decreases by approximately 4%. Notably, breastfeeding reduces the risk of hormone receptor–negative breast cancers, which are often more aggressive and less responsive to endocrine therapy.

10.4 Age at Menopause

Later age at natural menopause increases lifetime exposure to oestrogen.

Breast cancer risk increases by approximately 2.9% for each year of delay in natural menopause (Collaborative Group Meta-analysis, 2012).

Factors influencing later menopause include smoking cessation trends and widespread use of oral contraceptive pills. While menopause timing is not easily altered, awareness helps contextualise cumulative hormonal exposure.

10.5 Genetic Risk and Targeted Prevention

Genetics cannot be changed, but risk awareness can guide prevention.

While commercial gene panel testing may identify variants of uncertain significance, a small number of genes carry clearly established, high-penetrance risk.

BRCA1 and BRCA2

BRCA1 and BRCA2 are critical for DNA repair via homologous recombination. Pathogenic mutations substantially increase lifetime risk of:

- breast cancer,
- ovarian cancer,
- peritoneal cancer.

By age 70, breast cancer risk in BRCA mutation carriers approaches **65%**.

For individuals with:

- a strong family history of breast, ovarian, or peritoneal cancer,
- early-onset breast cancer in relatives, genetic counselling and testing may be appropriate.

Risk-Reduction Strategies for BRCA Carriers

Options include:

1. **Enhanced screening**
   - Initiation of annual breast MRI from approximately 25 years of age (MRI is more sensitive than mammography in young women with dense breast tissue).
2. **Risk-reducing surgery**
   - Prophylactic bilateral mastectomy, followed by reconstruction.
   - Prophylactic bilateral salpingo-oophorectomy after childbearing, which significantly reduces ovarian and breast cancer risk (USPSTF, 2019).

Other genes associated with increased risk, at varying magnitudes, include PALB2, TP53, ATM, CDH1, CHEK2, STK11, and PTEN. Each requires individualised risk assessment rather than blanket recommendations.

10.6 Screening: Detecting Cancer Early

Screening does not prevent breast cancer, but it prevents late detection, when treatment options are limited and outcomes poorer.

Screening Modalities

- Self-examination and clinical breast examination: limited sensitivity and prone to error.
- Mammography: the most effective population-level screening tool for early detection.

Early-stage detection:

- improves survival,
- reduces need for aggressive therapy,
- and improves quality of life.

Screening Recommendations (General Population)

- **United Kingdom**: mammography from 50–71 years.
- **United States**:

- o Annual screening from 45–54 years,
- o Biennial or continued annual screening from 55 years,
- o Optional early screening from 40 years.

High-Risk Individuals

Screening begins earlier and may involve MRI rather than mammography, particularly in those with:

- genetic predisposition,
- strong family history,
- prior chest radiation.

A critical reminder: men can also develop breast cancer, particularly in the presence of genetic risk factors.

A Precision-Based Conclusion

Breast cancer prevention is not about universal rules.
It is about timing, biology, and individual context.

Understanding hormonal exposure, reproductive history, genetic susceptibility, and screening options allows prevention to become personalised rather than generalised.

Precision prevention does not eliminate risk.
It shifts odds, often profoundly.

And in cancer, shifting odds matters.

Chapter 11

Precision Prevention of Colorectal Cancer

The room was quiet in the way procedure suites always are, efficient, impersonal, designed to minimise drama.

The patient lay on their side, mildly sedated, unaware that the most consequential moment of the day had already passed. On the monitor, the interior of the colon appeared in muted shades of pink and grey, folding and unfolding as the scope advanced. To the untrained eye, it looked unremarkable. Routine. Almost boring.

Then the polyp came into view.

Small. Pedunculated. Easily missed if one were not looking carefully enough. It had caused no pain, no bleeding, no warning. The patient had come in because the calendar said it was time, not because their body had asked for help.

With a practiced movement, the loop was positioned. A brief application of cautery. The polyp was removed, retrieved, and sent for histology. The screen returned to normal mucosa. The procedure continued.

From the patient's perspective, nothing had happened.

But biologically, everything had.

What had just been removed was not cancer. It was something far more important: a future cancer that never got the chance to exist.

Colorectal cancer does not appear suddenly. It evolves slowly, quietly, over years, sometimes decades, progressing step by step from benign cellular error to invasive malignancy. And unlike many cancers, this process leaves behind a visible, removable trail.

This is what makes colorectal cancer different.

And this is what makes it preventable.

Colorectal cancer is the third most commonly diagnosed cancer worldwide and remains a major cause of cancer-related mortality. Because it is frequently detected at advanced stages, it accounted for approximately 935,173 deaths globally in 2020 (IARC, 2018).

Yet among the cancers discussed in this book, colorectal cancer offers one of the widest and clearest margins for prevention.

11.1 Primary Prevention: Lowering Baseline Risk

The foundational risk factors for colorectal cancer overlap with those explored earlier: diet, physical activity, body weight, smoking, and alcohol consumption all exert meaningful influence over lifetime risk.

A diet rich in fibre supports gut motility and microbial diversity. Regular physical activity improves insulin sensitivity and reduces inflammation. Maintaining a healthy body weight limits chronic metabolic stress. Avoidance of smoking and moderation of alcohol reduce exposure to known carcinogens.

Beyond lifestyle, two nutrients deserve specific attention.

Calcium and Vitamin D

Long-term calcium intake has been consistently associated with a reduction in colorectal cancer risk. Importantly, this is not an immediate effect.

Data from the Nurses' Health Study indicate that meaningful risk reduction emerges only after approximately ten years of sustained calcium consumption at doses of around 1,000 mg per day (Zhang et al., 2016).

The biological mechanisms are plausible and complementary:

- calcium binds secondary bile acids that are toxic to the colonic epithelium,
- it neutralises haem iron and ionised fatty acids,
- and it reduces direct mucosal irritation that promotes chronic inflammation and malignant transformation (Gamage et al., 2018).

Vitamin D appears to act synergistically by supporting epithelial differentiation and immune regulation, although calcium remains the dominant factor in colorectal cancer prevention.

Prevention, here, is cumulative rather than dramatic, quiet biology reshaped over time.

11.2 Screening: Preventing Cancer by Removing Its Precursor

Screening is the cornerstone of colorectal cancer prevention.

Unlike many malignancies, colorectal cancer follows a predictable trajectory. Most cases arise from benign precursor lesions, most commonly adenomatous polyps, that gradually acquire malignant features over 10 to 15 years. This extended timeline creates a rare opportunity: cancer can be intercepted before it exists.

Screening Modalities

Several screening approaches are used worldwide:

- **Faecal occult blood testing** (**FOBT**) detects microscopic blood loss in stool.
- **Faecal immunochemical testing** (**FIT**) improves specificity by identifying human haemoglobin.
- **Colonoscopy** remains the gold standard.

Colonoscopy is unique in that it is both diagnostic and therapeutic. It allows direct visualisation of the colonic mucosa and immediate removal of adenomas before malignant transformation occurs.

Screening strategies vary by country:

- some regions employ FIT as a population-level screening tool,
- others rely primarily on colonoscopy.

For individuals at average risk, screening is typically recommended between 50 and 74 years of age, although guidelines continue to evolve as younger-onset disease becomes more common.

The power of screening lies not in detecting cancer early, but in preventing cancer altogether.

11.3 Genetic Syndromes and High-Risk Individuals

While most colorectal cancers are sporadic, a subset arises from inherited syndromes that dramatically increase lifetime risk. For these individuals, precision prevention is not optional, it is essential.

Lynch Syndrome (Hereditary Non-Polyposis Colorectal Cancer)

Lynch syndrome results from defects in DNA mismatch repair genes, leading to genomic instability. Affected individuals face a 60–80% lifetime risk of colorectal cancer.

In addition to colorectal cancer, Lynch syndrome increases the risk of:

- endometrial cancer,
- ovarian cancer,
- gastric cancer,
- pancreatic cancer,
- and other malignancies.

Screening colonoscopy is initiated earlier than in the general population, often before the age at which the youngest affected family member was diagnosed.

Familial Adenomatous Polyposis (FAP)

Familial adenomatous polyposis is characterised by the development of hundreds to thousands of adenomas, often beginning in adolescence. Without intervention, the risk of colorectal cancer approaches 100% by age 40.

Preventive management typically involves prophylactic colectomy, and in some cases removal of the rectum, tailored to disease burden and individual risk. Although FAP accounts for only about 1% of colorectal cancer cases (Patel et al., 2012), its implications are profound.

Who Should Seek Genetic Counselling

Individuals with:

- colorectal cancer in first-degree relatives,
- multiple affected family members,
- or diagnosis before the age of 50,

should consult healthcare professionals to assess the need for genetic counselling and personalised prevention strategies.

11.4 The Rising Threat of Young-Onset Colorectal Cancer

One of the most disturbing trends in modern oncology is the rising incidence of colorectal cancer among individuals aged 20 to 49 years. This pattern has been observed across multiple countries and cannot be dismissed as improved detection alone.

The causes are not fully understood, but several factors are strongly implicated:

- diets low in fibre and high in ultra-processed foods,
- depletion of beneficial gut microbiota,
- increased alcohol consumption,
- smoking,
- physical inactivity,
- prolonged sedentary behaviour, including excessive screen time.

This shift challenges long-held assumptions that colorectal cancer is a disease of older age and underscores the urgency of earlier awareness, symptom recognition, and risk assessment.

A Precision-Based Conclusion

Colorectal cancer exemplifies the promise of precision prevention.

- Long-term nutritional strategies can lower baseline risk.
- Screening can intercept cancer before it exists.
- Genetic insight can guide early, life-saving intervention.
- Lifestyle choices may counteract disturbing generational trends.

Few cancers offer such a wide margin for prevention.

In colorectal cancer, timing matters. Biology matters. Action matters.

And sometimes, prevention looks like nothing at all,
a quiet room,
a small polyp,
and a cancer that never gets the chance to exist.

Chapter 12

Precision Prevention of Melanoma

Opening Scene

The quad was unusually alive that afternoon.

It was one of those rare Oxford days when the sky holds its blue without apology and the sun lingers as if it belongs there. The rules about the grass, normally inviolate, had been relaxed for summer. Students lay scattered across the green, backpacks abandoned, faces turned upward, skin exposed in quiet celebration of warmth.

As I crossed the quad, a group of my medical students spotted me and waved, calling out my name with the easy familiarity that comes from shared classrooms and long terms. They were laughing, relaxed, unguarded.

What caught my attention was not their joy, but the light.

It was sharper than it felt. Unfiltered. The kind that does its work invisibly.

I smiled, waved back, and said something that landed awkwardly in the moment:
You should put some sunscreen on.

They laughed, good-naturedly. In England, sunlight feels like a gift too scarce to question. We miss it more than we fear it.

I kept walking.

The grass was cool underfoot. The sun stayed warm. Nothing happened.

That is how prevention usually works.

Ultraviolet radiation does not burn immediately. It does not announce damage as it accumulates. It writes itself quietly into DNA, one exposure at a time, remembered long after the warmth fades.

Melanoma begins like this:
not with pain,
not with alarm,
but with ordinary sunlight on ordinary skin.

Melanoma as a Preventable Cancer

Melanoma is an aggressive malignancy and accounts for a disproportionate number of skin cancer–related deaths worldwide. Its incidence has risen steadily across many countries, making it a growing public health concern.

Approximately 80% of melanomas are attributable to ultraviolet radiation (UVR) **from** excessive sun exposure.

While UV-independent mechanisms exist, particularly among highly susceptible individuals with red hair and fair skin (Mitra et al., 2012), from a prevention perspective, UV exposure remains the dominant and most modifiable risk factor.

Despite advances in therapy, more than 60,000 people die from melanoma globally each year (IARC). In England alone, the NHS spent over £180 million on skin cancers by 2020, underscoring the economic as well as human cost.

Melanoma is therefore a disease in which primary prevention can save lives, preserve quality of life, and reduce societal burden.

12.1 Biology of Melanoma and Skin Pigmentation

Melanomas arise from melanocytes, the pigment-producing cells of the skin. These cells synthesise melanin, which exists in two principal forms:

- **Eumelanin** (brown/black pigment), which provides substantial photoprotection against UV radiation
- **Pheomelanin** (red/yellow pigment), which offers far less UV protection and may itself contribute to oxidative stress

Human skin pigmentation evolved as an adaptive balance between UV protection and vitamin D synthesis.

- In regions with limited sunlight, lighter skin facilitated vitamin D production, reducing diseases such as rickets.
- In regions with intense sunlight, darker skin rich in eumelanin protected against UV-induced DNA damage.

Global migration disrupted this evolutionary balance. A striking example is Australia, where a predominantly fair-skinned population now lives under intense UV exposure, contributing to one of the highest melanoma rates in the world, particularly when contrasted with the native Aboriginal population.

12.2 Avoiding Excessive Ultraviolet Radiation

Melanoma risk accumulates slowly. So must its prevention.

The most effective strategy for melanoma prevention is limiting cumulative UV exposure, particularly during periods of peak intensity.

Key preventive measures include:

- Avoiding direct sun exposure during midday hours (typically 11 a.m. to 3 p.m.)

- Wearing wide-brimmed hats, UV-protective sunglasses, and protective clothing
- Using broad-spectrum sunscreen with SPF $\geq$ 30, containing agents such as avobenzone or titanium dioxide

Sunscreen should be:

- applied generously,
- reapplied every two hours,
- and reapplied after swimming or excessive sweating.

Importantly, sunscreen does not provide absolute protection. Seeking shade remains essential, even when sunscreen is used.

Environmental factors further complicate exposure:

- Snow can reflect up to 90% of UV radiation,
- UV exposure can occur even on overcast days (Kinney et al., 2000).

Childhood sun exposure deserves particular emphasis. Sunburns during childhood significantly increase the risk of melanoma and other skin cancers in adulthood (Dennis et al., 2008). Early education is therefore a cornerstone of precision prevention.

12.3 Avoiding Artificial Ultraviolet Exposure

Indoor tanning is not a safe alternative to sunlight.

Use of tanning beds and sunlamps is strongly associated with increased risk of:

- melanoma,
- basal cell carcinoma,
- squamous cell carcinoma (Wehner et al., 2012).

In addition to carcinogenesis, indoor tanning accelerates skin aging, causing wrinkles, loss of elasticity, and pigmentary changes (Quatresooz et al., 2011).

From a prevention standpoint, no level of indoor tanning is safe.

12.4 Why Sun Exposure Becomes Addictive

Ultraviolet-seeking behavior is not purely cultural, it has a biological basis.

UV radiation activates an endogenous opioid pathway. DNA damage caused by UV exposure triggers upregulation of proopiomelanocortin (POMC), which is subsequently cleaved into several peptides, including β-endorphin, the body's natural analgesic.

β-endorphin produces feelings of relaxation and reward, reinforcing UV-seeking behaviour and creating dependence on sun exposure or tanning beds (Lo et al., 2014).

This biology helps explain why harmful exposure often persists despite awareness of risk, and why prevention strategies must account for human neurobiology, not education alone.

12.5 Immune Surveillance and Melanoma Prevention

The immune system plays a central role in preventing melanoma development.

Effective immune surveillance enables recognition and elimination of melanocytes that have accumulated DNA damage. Factors that impair immune function weaken this protective capacity.

Conditions associated with increased melanoma risk include:

- HIV infection due to unprotected sexual practices,
- intravenous drug use,
- chronic immunosuppression (e.g., post-transplant therapy).

Individuals with compromised immune systems have a markedly increased risk of melanoma and other skin cancers, reinforcing the importance of immune health as part of a comprehensive prevention strategy.

A Precision-Based Conclusion

Melanoma is not inevitable.

Its risk is shaped by:

- skin pigmentation biology,
- cumulative UV exposure,
- childhood experiences,
- biologically reinforced behaviours,
- and immune competence.

Precision prevention of melanoma means recognising who is at risk, when exposure is most harmful, and which interventions are effective.

Avoiding excessive ultraviolet radiation, natural or artificial, remains the single most powerful preventive measure. Combined with immune health and early education, this approach can dramatically reduce melanoma incidence.

In melanoma, prevention is not subtle.
It is visible.
It is actionable.

And when it works
nothing happens.

Chapter 13

Precision Prevention of Liver Cancer

The scan was already on the screen when I walked into the room.

A familiar grayscale, liver margins outlined too clearly, too irregularly. The kind of image that announces itself before anyone speaks. The room was quiet in that peculiar way examination rooms become when no one wants to be the first to break the silence.

The patient sat upright, hands folded in his lap. His eyes were not on the monitor, but on the wall behind it, as if distance might soften what was about to be said.

He had come in feeling well.

No pain. No jaundice. No fatigue that would have raised concern. The blood tests had been ordered almost casually, routine, preventative, something to be checked before the next appointment. The abnormality had surprised everyone. Including him.

When I asked about his history, the story unfolded slowly. He had been born in a country where childhood vaccination was not routine at the time. His mother remembered an illness when he was an infant, nothing dramatic, no hospital admission, just a fever that passed.

He had never thought about it again.

For decades, neither had his liver.

A vaccine he never received.
An infection he never knew he carried.
An organ that compensated faithfully, until it could not.

That is how hepatocellular carcinoma often announces itself: not with drama, but with delay.

Liver cancer rarely begins as cancer. It begins as injury, sustained quietly over years. Viral. Toxic. Inflammatory. By the time a mass appears on a scan, the biological process has often been underway longer than most people can remember.

What struck me in that room was not only the diagnosis, but how avoidable the path to it had been.

Liver cancer, more than most malignancies, tells its story backward. To understand how it appears, one must trace it to exposures that occurred decades earlier, often in childhood, often invisibly. And in doing so, one encounters a rare clarity in oncology: a cancer whose major causes are known, measurable, and interruptible.

It is here that precision prevention is not a theory, but a practice.

Liver cancer is among the leading causes of cancer-related mortality worldwide. The most common form, hepatocellular carcinoma (HCC), almost always arises on a background of chronic liver injury and inflammation.

Unlike many cancers, liver cancer is frequently the end result of identifiable, preventable exposures. Precision prevention therefore focuses on interrupting these causal pathways early, long before malignant transformation occurs.

13.1 Hepatitis B Virus and Liver Cancer

Chronic infection with Hepatitis B virus (HBV) is one of the strongest known risk factors for hepatocellular carcinoma.

HBV can be transmitted:

- from mother to child at birth,
- through close household contact,
- via blood or bodily fluids.

When infection occurs early in life, particularly during infancy, the likelihood of developing chronic hepatitis is high. Chronic HBV infection leads to persistent inflammation, progressive liver damage, cirrhosis, and eventually hepatocellular carcinoma.

Hepatitis B Vaccination: A Cancer-Preventing Vaccine

Hepatitis B vaccination is one of the most effective cancer-prevention strategies in modern medicine.

When administered appropriately and in the absence of contraindications, HBV vaccination dramatically reduces the risk of chronic infection, and by extension, liver cancer.

Population-level success stories provide compelling evidence:

- In Taiwan, universal vaccination introduced in 1982 led to a marked reduction in childhood and adult hepatocellular carcinoma.
- Similar declines were observed in Thailand from 1988 onward and among Indigenous populations in Alaska.

These outcomes represent one of the clearest demonstrations in modern medicine that vaccination can prevent cancer.

From a precision-prevention standpoint, universal hepatitis B vaccination remains essential.

13.2 Hepatitis C Virus: A Silent Carcinogen

Hepatitis C virus (HCV) is a common blood-borne pathogen and a major contributor to liver cancer worldwide. Unlike HBV, there is currently no vaccine against HCV.

Chronic HCV infection is associated not only with hepatocellular carcinoma, but also with non-Hodgkin's lymphoma.

A major challenge is that approximately 80% of infected individuals are asymptomatic, allowing the infection to progress silently for decades. In 2015, more than 70 million people worldwide were living with chronic HCV infection (WHO, 2016).

Risk Factors and Prevention

HCV transmission occurs primarily through exposure to infected blood, including:

- sharing needles among intravenous drug users,
- unsafe tattooing or body piercing,
- unregulated acupuncture practices,
- unprotected sexual contact.

Precision prevention relies on early identification and treatment, particularly in high-risk populations. Modern antiviral therapies can eradicate HCV, halting chronic inflammation and substantially reducing future cancer risk.

Avoidance of blood exposure and proactive testing are therefore critical components of liver-cancer prevention.

13.3 Aflatoxin: An Environmental Carcinogen

Not all liver carcinogens are viral.

In the early 1960s, a mysterious outbreak known as "Turkey X disease" killed more than 100,000 turkeys in England. The cause was later identified as aflatoxin, a toxic by-product of the fungus *Aspergillus flavus*, which had contaminated imported feed from Brazil.

Aflatoxin is:

- odourless,
- tasteless,
- and easily ingested unknowingly.

Among its variants, aflatoxin B1 is particularly potent and has been classified by the International Agency for Research on Cancer (IARC) as causally linked to hepatocellular carcinoma.

Mechanism of Carcinogenesis

Aflatoxin causes direct DNA damage and induces characteristic mutations in the tumour-suppressor gene p53, a key guardian against malignant transformation. This molecular signature has been repeatedly observed in liver cancers arising in regions with high aflatoxin exposure.

Aflatoxin contamination is most common in:

- warm, humid climates,
- regions with inadequate food-storage infrastructure.

Crops at risk include:

- maize,
- wheat,
- rice,
- beans,
- nuts, particularly peanuts.

While many developed nations enforce strict regulatory limits, exposure remains a significant risk in parts of the developing world. Travelers should remain mindful of food safety standards when visiting regions with limited regulation.

13.4 Alcohol and Industrial Toxins

In addition to viral and fungal exposures, environmental toxins significantly contribute to liver-cancer risk.

Chronic alcohol consumption induces liver inflammation, fibrosis, and cirrhosis, conditions that dramatically increase the likelihood of hepatocellular carcinoma.

Other industrial toxins, such as vinyl chloride, are also established liver carcinogens, particularly among exposed workers.

A Precision-Based Conclusion

Liver cancer exemplifies the power of precision prevention.

- **Hepatitis B vaccination** can prevent cancer decades before it would otherwise appear.
- **Early detection and treatment of Hepatitis C** can interrupt a silent progression toward malignancy.
- **Avoidance of aflatoxin-contaminated food and environmental toxins** reduces genomic injury at its source.
- **Alcohol moderation** protects the liver's regenerative capacity.

Few cancers offer such clearly defined opportunities for prevention.

In liver cancer, the right intervention, applied early, to the right individual, can mean the difference between irreversible disease and a lifetime without it.

Precision prevention, here, is not aspirational.
It is proven.

Chapter 14

Precision Prevention: Cervical Cancer

The room is small, quiet, and deliberately neutral.

A paper sheet rustles as it is unfolded. A plastic speculum clicks into place. The woman on the examination table stares at the ceiling, counting the faint stains in the acoustic tiles, not from fear, but from habit. This is routine. It is supposed to be.

Outside the room, life continues uninterrupted. Phones vibrate. Appointments run late. Someone laughs down the corridor.

Inside, a few cells are gently brushed from the surface of the cervix, cells that look identical to millions of others, indistinguishable to the naked eye. They will be dropped into liquid, labelled, and sent away.

No pain.
No drama.
No sense that anything consequential has occurred.

And yet, if something is wrong, this is the moment it can still be stopped.

Not treated.
Stopped.

Years later, if cancer is prevented, nothing will mark this
visit as extraordinary. There will be no scar, no story, no
anniversary. The success of this moment will be measured
entirely by its absence, by a disease that never arrives.

That is the paradox of prevention.
When it works, it disappears.

Only now do we widen the lens.

Cervical cancer, more than almost any other malignancy,
exposes this truth. It is not a sudden betrayal of the body,
nor a mystery written into fate. It is a process, slow,
detectable, and, in most cases, avoidable.

What determines the outcome is not luck, but timing.
Not heroics, but access.
Not treatment, but interception.

Cervical cancer remains one of the most common cancers
affecting women worldwide. Yet unlike many malignancies,
it is almost entirely preventable.

Nearly all cases arise from persistent infection with two
oncogenic strains of the human papillomavirus (HPV),
types 16 and 18. Because HPV is sexually transmitted,
cervical cancer represents one of the clearest examples of a

malignancy in which biology, behaviour, vaccination, and screening intersect decisively.

Precision prevention of cervical cancer rests on two complementary pillars:

1. **Vaccination**, which prevents infection with high-risk HPV strains.
2. **Screening**, which detects precursor lesions early enough to prevent progression to invasive disease.

When both are used appropriately, protection against cervical cancer is exceptionally high.

14.1 Screening: Intercepting Cancer Before It Exists

The introduction of cervical screening transformed women's health.

Cervical cancer does not emerge overnight. It develops slowly, progressing over years from precancerous lesions to invasive carcinoma. This prolonged latent period creates a rare opportunity in oncology: the chance to intervene before cancer exists at all, provided abnormal cells are detected early.

The Pap Smear: A Revolutionary Test

The Pap smear is named after George Nicholas Papanicolaou, a Greek physician whose path to medicine was anything but linear. Initially trained in the humanities and music, he entered medicine at the insistence of his physician father. He later earned a PhD in zoology from the University of Munich by 1910.

In 1913, Papanicolaou emigrated to the United States with his wife, carrying just 250 dollars. For a year, he worked multiple jobs, including selling rugs and playing the violin, before securing a position in the pathology department at New York University. He later became an assistant professor at Cornell University.

His work was influenced by earlier ideas from British physician Walter Hayle Walshe, who had proposed in the 19th century that cancerous cells could be identified microscopically. In parallel, Aurel Babeș, a Romanian physician, demonstrated in 1927 that malignant cells could be detected by sampling cervical cells using a platinum loop.

Yet it was Papanicolaou's refinement of technique, and perhaps the scientific ecosystem in which he worked, that led to widespread adoption of the method now known as the Pap smear.

In 1943, alongside gynaecologist Dr. Herbert Traut, Papanicolaou published *Diagnosis of Uterine Cancer by the Vaginal Smear*. Early methods were crude, involving collection of vaginal fluid using glass pipettes. In 1947, Canadian gynaecologist J. Ernest Ayre introduced the Ayre spatula, significantly improving sample collection (Ayre et al., 1947).

Modern techniques have evolved far beyond these early methods, but the principle remains unchanged:

Early detection saves lives, by preventing cancer from ever forming.

Screening Recommendations

Because cervical cancer progresses slowly, regular screening is highly effective:

- Pap smear testing every 3 years for women aged 25–49
- Every 5 years for women aged 50–64
- Increasingly, HPV testing, used alone or in combination with cytology

Screening does not merely detect cancer early.
It prevents cancer altogether by identifying and treating precursor lesions.

14.2 Human Papillomavirus and the Biology of Prevention

The causal link between HPV and cervical cancer was established in the early 1980s.

In 1983, **Harald Zur Hausen**, along with **Lutz Gissmann**, demonstrated that HPV infection was central to cervical carcinogenesis, a discovery that fundamentally altered cancer biology and later earned Zur Hausen the Nobel Prize.

Subsequent molecular mechanisms were elucidated by scientists including **Professor Peter M. Howley**, whose work clarified how high-risk HPV oncoproteins disrupt tumour-suppressor pathways, driving malignant transformation.

14.3 The HPV Vaccine: Preventing Cancer at Its Root

The development of the HPV vaccine represents one of the most important advances in cancer prevention.

Dr. Ian H. Frazer, a Scottish clinician-scientist working in Australia, became deeply interested in HPV after a brief encounter with Harald Zur Hausen in Germany. Alongside **Dr. Jian Zhou** at the University of Queensland,

Frazer developed virus-like particle technology that formed the basis of the HPV vaccine.

A subsequent legal dispute over intellectual priority was ultimately resolved in favour of Frazer and Zhou, tragically after Dr. Zhou had passed away.

The HPV vaccine has since been shown to be highly effective in preventing infection with oncogenic HPV strains and, by extension, cervical cancer.

Vaccination Strategy

For maximum efficacy, HPV vaccination should occur before sexual debut.

In England, the NHS administers the HPV vaccine to both boys and girls aged 12–13 years, reflecting an understanding that:

- HPV affects all sexes
- herd immunity enhances protection
- prevention should be equitable and universal

Interlude: The lecture hall

The room was quiet in the way lecture halls become when something important is about to be said.

It was at Harvard, one of those windowless rooms where attention narrows and time compresses. **Peter Howley** stood at the front, not speaking about cancer as a disease, but about a virus as a strategy.

He wrote two symbols on the board:

E6
E7

There was nothing theatrical about the moment. No announcement that this was the key. But as the lecture unfolded, it became clear that these two proteins explained something that had long resisted clarity.

Certain human papillomaviruses, particularly types 16 and 18, did not merely infect cells. They reprogrammed them.

E6 dismantled *p53*, the cell's final checkpoint.
E7 neutralised *Rb*, releasing the brakes on proliferation.

Cancer, in this framing, was not a sudden catastrophe. It was a maintained state, sustained by the continued expression of viral machinery.

Remove the machinery, and the system could recover. Prevent the infection, and the cancer would never arise.

I remember thinking, not for the first time, that prevention often begins as a molecular insight no one yet knows how to use.

Years later, in another lecture, this time by John Schiller from the National Cancer Institute, that insight had become an intervention.

Schiller spoke about virus-like particles: structures that looked enough like HPV to train the immune system, yet carried no genetic material and posed no risk. The elegance of it was unmistakable, teach the body to recognise the virus *before* it ever learned how to hide.

Toward the end of the talk, he mentioned, almost casually, that his daughter had received the HPV vaccine.

The room did not change.
No one applauded.

But the meaning of the science shifted.

What had begun as E6 and E7 on a blackboard had ended as a choice made at a kitchen table.

Between those two rooms, separated by years and disciplines, a preventable cancer had quietly become optional.

14.4 A Preventable Cancer

Cervical cancer stands apart.

- It is caused by a known virus.
- That virus can be prevented by vaccination.
- Its precursor lesions can be detected and treated.
- Its progression is slow enough to allow interception.

Practicing safe sex, receiving HPV vaccination, and
adhering to routine screening schedules together
provide near-complete protection against cervical cancer.

A Precision-Based Conclusion

Cervical cancer is not a failure of biology.
It is a failure of access, awareness, or adherence.

Precision prevention offers a different outcome, one in
which the right intervention, delivered at the right time,
eliminates disease before it begins.

Few cancers offer such clarity.
Fewer still offer such hope.

Cervical cancer belongs to the latter.

Chapter 15

Precision Prevention of Prostate Cancer

The man sat across from me, hands folded, eyes fixed on the floor rather than on the scan between us.

He was not old. Not by any intuitive measure. He spoke carefully, as if choosing words that would not betray how unexpected this moment felt. He had come in for what he assumed would be reassurance, routine tests, mild urinary symptoms, nothing dramatic. Prostate cancer, in his mind, belonged to a later decade of life, something distant and theoretical.

When the diagnosis was spoken aloud, it landed quietly. No collapse. No anger. Just a pause long enough to reveal the recalibration happening inside him.

His first question was not about treatment.

It was about *why*.

He had never smoked. He exercised. He had no striking family history. He wanted to know what he had done wrong, or what he had failed to do.

That question is the most common one men ask when faced with prostate cancer. And it is also the most difficult to answer honestly.

Because prostate cancer rarely offers a single culprit. It does not announce itself as the consequence of one habit or one exposure. Instead, it accumulates, slowly, silently, at the intersection of time, hormones, inflammation, genetics, and the ordinary biological rhythms of life.

What matters, I realised yet again, is not blame, but pattern.

And pattern is where precision prevention begins.

Prostate cancer is the second most commonly diagnosed cancer among men worldwide and a leading cause of cancer-related mortality. In 2018 alone, approximately 359,000 men died from prostate cancer globally (Ferlay et al., 2018).

Unlike cancers driven predominantly by a single exposure, prostate cancer arises from a complex interplay of age, hormones, inflammation, genetics, and lifestyle factors. Precision prevention therefore focuses on identifying modifiable biological pathways rather than assigning simple causes.

15.1 Infection, Inflammation, and Cancer Risk

Several cancers discussed in earlier chapters demonstrate clear links between chronic infection and malignancy, including:

- human papillomavirus and cervical cancer,
- hepatitis B virus and liver cancer,
- Epstein–Barr virus and certain lymphomas,
- Merkel cell polyomavirus and skin cancer.

These examples highlight a broader principle: persistent inflammation, regardless of its source, can create a tissue environment conducive to carcinogenesis.

The prostate gland is particularly susceptible to inflammatory insults. Chronic prostatitis and inflammatory infiltrates are frequently observed in prostate tissue and have been proposed as contributors to malignant transformation through oxidative stress, DNA damage, and altered immune surveillance.

15.2 Ejaculatory Frequency and Prostate Cancer Risk

An unexpected but increasingly studied factor in prostate cancer prevention is ejaculatory frequency.

A large prospective cohort study conducted in the United States followed 31,925 male health professionals over nearly 18 years. The study reported that men with higher ejaculatory frequency during young adulthood had a significantly reduced risk of developing prostate cancer later in life (Rider et al., 2016).

These findings were later supported by data from Australia, where prostate cancer contributes disproportionately to male cancer mortality.

Proposed Biological Mechanisms

Several hypotheses may explain this association:

- regular ejaculation may reduce prostatic fluid stasis, limiting accumulation of carcinogenic secretions,
- it may decrease chronic inflammation within the prostate,
- and it may reduce exposure of prostatic epithelium to oxidative stress.

Importantly, these studies demonstrate association, not causation, and do not imply that sexual behaviour alone determines cancer risk. Rather, they suggest that normal physiological clearance mechanisms may play a protective role.

15.3 Precision Prevention, Not Prescription

It is neither appropriate nor necessary to medicalise intimacy. The relevance of these findings lies not in behavioural instruction, but in biological insight.

Prostate cancer risk appears to be influenced by:

- hormonal dynamics,
- inflammatory burden,
- and tissue homeostasis over decades.

Understanding these mechanisms may, in the future, inform risk stratification, counselling, and individualised prevention strategies, particularly for men at elevated baseline risk.

A Precision-Based Conclusion

Prostate cancer prevention does not hinge on a single action or exposure. It emerges from maintaining physiological balance, minimising chronic inflammation, and supporting long-term tissue health.

Large cohort studies remind us that everyday biological processes, often overlooked, may influence cancer risk in subtle but meaningful ways.

Precision prevention is not about prescribing lifestyles. It is about recognising patterns, understanding mechanisms, and using evidence to shift risk.

In prostate cancer, as in much of oncology, small biological advantages accumulated over time can matter profoundly.

Chapter 16

Precision Prevention: Environmental Risk Factors

The glass was already full when I noticed the hesitation.

It was an ordinary moment: a tap turned, water catching the light, a reflexive reach for a glass. The water was clear. No smell. No discoloration. It tasted exactly as water should, of nothing at all.

And yet, I paused.

Not because there was anything visibly wrong, but because experience had taught me something uncomfortable: the most dangerous exposures rarely announce themselves.

They do not burn.
They do not sting.
They do not warn.

They enter quietly, through a sip, a breath, a habit repeated daily, accumulating not as symptoms, but as probability.

By the time disease appears, the exposure has usually done its work.

We tend to imagine environmental risk as something distant: a polluted river elsewhere, a factory someone else lives beside, a problem confined to places without regulation or resources. But exposure does not respect geography, income, or intention. It flows through pipes, settles in soil, concentrates in enclosed spaces, and persists long after its source has faded from view.

That is what makes environmental carcinogens uniquely insidious.

They do not require consent.
They do not depend on behaviour.
They enter through the most essential acts of living, drinking water, breathing air, inhabiting shelter.

Precision prevention, therefore, cannot stop at personal choice. It must extend outward, to the environments we trust without question, and to the systems that shape what enters our bodies long before we are aware of it.

16.1 Drinking Water: An Invisible Exposure

Nearly 60% of the adult human body is water. Cellular metabolism, detoxification, and DNA repair all depend on it. Yet access to truly safe drinking water, one of the most basic prerequisites for health, is increasingly compromised.

It is tempting to assume water contamination is a problem confined to low-income nations. In reality, it is global.

New Zealand offers a sobering example.

A country associated with glaciers, open pasture, and environmental purity underwent a rapid agricultural shift from sheep farming to intensive dairy production. Increased cattle density demanded greater use of synthetic nitrogen fertilisers. The consequence was a sharp rise in nitrate concentrations in rivers and groundwater.

Elevated nitrates promote toxic algal blooms and bacterial overgrowth, rendering lakes unsafe even for recreational use. More importantly, chronic nitrate ingestion increases cancer risk, particularly colorectal cancer, through the formation of carcinogenic *N-nitroso compounds* in the gut.

The exposure is silent. The effect is cumulative.

16.2 PFAS: Persistent Chemicals, Persistent Risk

If nitrates represent contamination we can sometimes measure and regulate, PFAS represent exposure that persists even after the source disappears.

Polyfluoroalkyl and perfluoroalkyl substances, often called *"forever chemicals"*, are widely used in industrial processes, firefighting foams, food packaging, and non-stick coatings. They resist degradation, bioaccumulate, and circulate globally.

PFAS exposure has been shown to:

- impair immune function,
- disrupt endocrine signalling,
- and reduce vaccine responsiveness.

A landmark Danish study of adolescents from the Faroe Islands demonstrated that early-life PFAS exposure significantly diminished immune response (Grandjean et al., 2017). A compromised immune system weakens one of the body's most critical defenses against cancer: immune surveillance.

In parts of the United States, PFAS concentrations in drinking water exceed recommended safety thresholds by more than 190-fold (EPA, 2016).

16.3 Heavy Metals in Foods We Trust

Environmental exposure does not end at the tap.

Even foods associated with pleasure, quality, and well-being can serve as vectors for contamination. In recent independent analyses, dark chocolate products, including premium brands, were found to contain measurable levels of lead and cadmium.

These metals do not originate in the chocolate-making process itself. They enter through contaminated soil, accumulate in cacao plants, and persist through processing.

Both lead and cadmium are well-established toxicants, capable of interfering with DNA repair, immune function, and cellular signalling when exposure is chronic.

Occasional consumption is unlikely to confer meaningful cancer risk. But the finding illustrates a broader principle of precision prevention:

Exposure is rarely dramatic. It is cumulative.

Cancer risk is shaped not by a single indulgence, but by the quiet addition of low-level toxicants over decades, often through sources we never suspect.

This is not a call for fear. It is a call for awareness.

16.4 Arsenic and Synergistic Carcinogenesis

Arsenic contamination remains a major global hazard, particularly in groundwater. It is a well-established carcinogen linked to cancers of the skin, lung, bladder, and liver.

But environmental carcinogenesis is rarely linear.

Risk is often synergistic.

Arsenic exposure combined with benzo(a)pyrene, a carcinogen encountered through cigarette smoke or charred meat, dramatically amplifies cancer risk (Zhishan et al., 2020). Each exposure alone may appear modest; together, they accelerate malignant transformation.

Precision prevention requires recognising how multiple low-level exposures interact, not merely tallying them in isolation.

16.5 Environmental Justice and Unequal Exposure

Economic growth and public health should not be opposing forces.

Those with resources can purchase filtered water, controlled air, and safer housing. Others rely entirely on what flows from aging infrastructure or surrounds industrial zones and agricultural runoff.

Environmental exposure is not evenly distributed, and cancer risk follows the same pattern.

Precision prevention therefore includes advocacy and accountability, not just individual vigilance.

16.6 Radon: The Air Inside Our Homes

Water is not the only invisible exposure.

Radon is a naturally occurring radioactive gas produced by the decay of uranium in the Earth's crust. It is colourless, odourless, tasteless, and highly carcinogenic.

Radon accumulates in enclosed spaces, particularly basements and ground-level rooms. As it decays, it releases alpha particles capable of inducing DNA damage.

Unusually high lung cancer rates among miners in Eastern Europe were reported as early as 1879. By 1929, radon was identified as the cause. In 1988, the International Agency for Research on Cancer formally classified radon as a carcinogen.

16.7 Radon Risk and Mitigation

Large epidemiological studies from Europe, the United States, and China demonstrate that even residential radon exposure increases lung cancer risk, particularly among smokers.

Radon contributes to:

- ~8% of lung cancer deaths in Europe,
- ~22,000 deaths annually in the United States,
- ~3.3% of lung cancer deaths in the UK.

Radon enters homes through:

- foundation cracks,
- gaps around pipes,
- porous building materials,
- crawl spaces and basements.

Mitigation strategies are effective and include:

- soil depressurisation systems,
- improved ventilation,
- sealed foundations.

Testing kits are inexpensive and widely available.
Awareness alone can prevent thousands of deaths.

A Precision-Based Conclusion

Environmental carcinogens challenge the notion that
cancer risk is solely a matter of personal choice.

Precision prevention recognises that:

- exposures are unevenly distributed,
- risks accumulate silently,
- and prevention often requires structural solutions,
  not just willpower.

Clean water and safe air are not luxuries.
They are biological prerequisites.

Environmental awareness is not alarmism.
It is realism.

And realism, applied early, saves lives.

Chapter 17

Precision Prevention: Infections Beyond HPV and Hepatitis

The first time I saw it, there was nothing remarkable about the complaint.

The patient was middle-aged, otherwise healthy, sitting upright on the examination couch. He spoke of vague abdominal discomfort, nothing severe enough to worry him, no weight loss, no bleeding. Just a sense, he said, that something had never quite settled.

He had grown up elsewhere. A different country. A different childhood. He remembered bouts of stomach trouble when he was young, nothing dramatic, nothing treated. Time had carried him forward, as it does most of us, without ceremony.

The tests came back slowly.
Routine at first.
Then less so.

When the biopsy results arrived, they told a story that had begun decades earlier.

Not with a mutation, but with a guest.

Spiral-shaped. Microscopic. Persistent.

A bacterium that had arrived quietly, inflamed tissue patiently, and rewritten cellular behaviour over years rather than weeks.

Cancer, in this case, was not a sudden betrayal of the body.

It was the long memory of an infection never cleared.

Only later, after the diagnosis, after the treatment plans, did the larger realisation settle in. This cancer was not rare. It was not mysterious. And it was not inevitable.

It was preventable.

What followed was not an isolated lesson, but a pattern repeated across continents and conditions: viruses that persist, parasites that embed, immune systems slowly eroded. In each case, malignancy did not emerge from chaos, but from duration.

Cancer, I learned, does not always begin with a genetic accident.

Sometimes, it begins with something we once called ordinary.

17.1 Chronic Infection as a Carcinogenic State

Not all cancers arise from mutations alone. In a significant fraction of cases, malignancy emerges as the late consequence of chronic infection, persistent inflammation, and prolonged immune activation.

The recognition that microbes can cause cancer was once controversial. Today, it is firmly established that approximately 15–20% of cancers worldwide are infection-associated, with a disproportionate burden in low- and middle-income countries. Crucially, many of these cancers are preventable.

Acute infections are rarely carcinogenic. Chronicity is what matters.

Persistent infections can:

- induce long-standing inflammation,
- generate reactive oxygen and nitrogen species,
- impair DNA repair,
- alter epigenetic regulation,
- and distort immune surveillance.

Over time, these processes create a microenvironment conducive to malignant transformation.

17.2 *Helicobacter pylori* and Gastric Cancer

Helicobacter pylori is a spiral-shaped bacterium that colonises the stomach and infects nearly half of the global population.

While most infected individuals remain asymptomatic, chronic infection can lead to:

- atrophic gastritis,
- intestinal metaplasia,
- dysplasia,
- and ultimately gastric adenocarcinoma.

Certain strains expressing the CagA virulence factor are particularly oncogenic, disrupting cellular signalling and promoting genomic instability.

The World Health Organisation classifies *H. pylori* as a Group 1 carcinogen.

Precision Prevention

- Testing and eradication with antibiotics significantly reduces gastric cancer risk
- Population-level screening shows benefit in high-incidence regions
- High-salt diets, smoked foods, and smoking synergise with infection to increase risk

17.3 Epstein-Barr Virus (EBV): A Ubiquitous Virus with Selective Consequences

Epstein–Barr virus infects more than 90% of humans worldwide, usually during childhood or adolescence.

In most individuals, the virus remains latent and harmless. However, EBV is causally linked to:

- Hodgkin lymphoma,
- Burkitt lymphoma,
- nasopharyngeal carcinoma,
- certain gastric cancers,
- and post-transplant lymphoproliferative disorders.

EBV-driven cancers arise through viral proteins that:

- promote cell survival,
- inhibit apoptosis,
- and evade immune detection.

Precision Prevention

- There is currently no licensed EBV vaccine
- Risk is highest in settings of immune suppression
- Early recognition and immune reconstitution are critical preventive strategies

17.4 Schistosomiasis and Bladder Cancer

In regions where parasitic infections remain endemic, schistosomiasis is a major but underappreciated carcinogenic exposure.

Schistosoma haematobium deposits eggs in the bladder wall, leading to:

- chronic inflammation,
- fibrosis,
- squamous metaplasia,
- and squamous cell carcinoma of the bladder.

This association represents one of the earliest recognised links between infection and cancer.

Precision Prevention

- Sanitation and safe water access
- Anti-parasitic treatment programs
- Vector control

These interventions dramatically reduce cancer incidence at the population level.

17.5 HIV: Cancer Risk Through Immune Suppression

Human immunodeficiency virus does not directly cause cancer. Instead, it disables immune surveillance, allowing oncogenic viruses and transformed cells to escape detection.

HIV infection is associated with increased risk of:

- Kaposi sarcoma (HHV-8),
- non-Hodgkin lymphoma,
- cervical and anal cancers,
- hepatocellular carcinoma.

Antiretroviral therapy has substantially reduced, but not eliminated, these risks.

Precision Prevention

- Early diagnosis and sustained viral suppression
- HPV and hepatitis vaccination
- Regular cancer screening in high-risk populations

17.6 A Preventable Fraction

What unites these infections is not inevitability, but opportunity.

Unlike inherited mutations, infection-associated cancers offer multiple points of intervention:

- vaccination,
- antimicrobial treatment,
- sanitation,
- screening,
- immune preservation.

The success of **HPV** and hepatitis **B** vaccination programs demonstrates what is possible when biology, policy, and prevention align.

A Precision-Based Conclusion

Cancer prevention is not limited to lifestyle choices or genetic destiny. In many cases, it depends on recognising, and interrupting, long-standing biological insults.

Chronic infection is one such insult.

By identifying high-risk pathogens, treating them early, and preventing transmission, we can eliminate entire categories of cancer before they begin.

Infection-associated cancers remind us of a central truth of precision prevention:

Some cancers are not merely treatable.
They are avoidable.

Chapter 18

Early Symptoms People Ignore

It began, as these things often do, with something small.

A trace of blood on toilet paper. Not enough to alarm. Not enough to mention. It appeared once, then disappeared, then returned weeks later. He told himself it was haemorrhoids. He sat too long at work. He hadn't been drinking enough water. Everyone has something like this, he thought.

Life moved on.

There were meetings to attend, children to collect, emails that demanded immediate replies. The body, after all, is expected to endure. And when it does not protest loudly, we assume it is coping.

Months passed.

He noticed he was tired more often. Not exhausted, just a little less himself. He blamed age. Stress. Poor sleep. When his trousers loosened, he felt a brief flicker of satisfaction before explaining it away as skipped meals and long days.

The blood appeared again, faint and intermittent. He googled it once, late at night, scrolling until reassurance surfaced. The internet is generous with benign explanations.

He did not tell his partner.
He did not tell his doctor.

By the time pain arrived, it was no longer subtle.
By the time he sought help, the disease had already moved beyond where it began, quietly, efficiently, without drama.

What haunted him later was not that the cancer had been aggressive.

It was that it had been polite.

One of the most tragic aspects of cancer is not that it can be aggressive, but that it is often quiet at the beginning.

Many cancers announce themselves subtly, through symptoms that are easy to dismiss, normalise, or rationalise. By the time they become impossible to ignore, the disease may already have advanced beyond its site of origin. Early recognition does not guarantee cure, but **delay almost guarantees lost opportunity**.

This chapter is not meant to provoke fear.
It is meant to cultivate attentiveness.

18.1 Why Early Symptoms Are Overlooked

Early warning signs are often ignored not because people are careless, but because they are human.

Symptoms are dismissed when:

- they are intermittent or painless,
- they resemble benign conditions,
- embarrassment delays disclosure,
- caregiving roles take precedence over self-care,
- reassurance is sought from the internet rather than a physician.

In modern life, distraction is often mistaken for resilience.

18.2 Gastrointestinal Symptoms

Rectal bleeding

Rectal bleeding is frequently attributed to haemorrhoids. While haemorrhoids are common, rectal bleeding should never be automatically assumed to be benign, particularly:

- after the age of 40,
- when associated with weight loss, anaemia, or changes in bowel habits.

Colorectal cancer often develops slowly and is highly preventable when detected early.

Persistent change in bowel habits

New-onset constipation or diarrhoea, change in stool calibre, or a persistent feeling of incomplete evacuation, especially when lasting more than a few weeks, warrants medical evaluation.

Difficulty swallowing (dysphagia)

Progressive difficulty swallowing, first solids and later liquids, can signal oesophageal cancer. This symptom is often ignored until eating becomes impossible. Early-stage disease is far more amenable to curative treatment.

18.3 Unexplained Weight Loss and Fatigue

Unintentional weight loss is often celebrated or ignored.

When weight loss occurs without dietary change or increased activity, it should be taken seriously.

Similarly, fatigue that does not improve with rest, particularly when accompanied by pallor or shortness of breath, may reflect anaemia from occult blood loss or systemic disease.

18.4 Gynaecological Symptoms

Postmenopausal bleeding

Any bleeding after menopause is abnormal until proven otherwise and must be evaluated promptly. It can be an early sign of endometrial or cervical cancer.

Abnormal vaginal bleeding or discharge

Bleeding between periods, bleeding after intercourse, or unusual discharge should never be normalised, especially in women who have missed routine screening.

Women's symptoms are disproportionately minimised, by society and often by women themselves.

18.5 Breast Changes Beyond Lumps

Breast cancer does not always present as a lump.

Other warning signs include:

- skin dimpling or puckering,
- nipple retraction,
- spontaneous nipple discharge,
- redness or a peau d'orange appearance.

Pain is not a reliable discriminator between benign and malignant breast disease.

18.6 Skin Changes

Skin cancers are often visible, yet ignored.

Warning signs include:

- new pigmented lesions,
- changes in size, shape, or colour of an existing mole,
- irregular borders or bleeding,
- lesions that itch, crust, or fail to heal.

The ABCDE rule, Asymmetry, Border, Colour, Diameter, Evolving, remains a simple and effective guide.

18.7 Persistent Lumps and Swellings

Any lump that:

- persists beyond a few weeks,
- grows progressively,
- or feels hard or fixed,

requires assessment.

This includes lymph nodes in the neck, armpit, or groin, as well as testicular masses, which are often painless and highly curable when detected early.

18.8 Respiratory and Voice Changes

A cough lasting more than three weeks, persistent hoarseness, or coughing up blood, particularly in smokers or former smokers, should never be ignored.

Early lung and laryngeal cancers may present subtly.

18.9 Pain That Persists

Cancer-related pain is often late, but persistent, unexplained pain, particularly bone pain, headaches with neurological symptoms, or abdominal pain with weight loss, requires investigation.

Pain should not be endured as a badge of resilience.

18.10 The Cost of Delay

Cancer outcomes are strongly stage-dependent.

Early-stage disease often allows:

- less aggressive treatment,
- preservation of organ function,
- better quality of life,
- higher survival rates.

Delay converts potentially curable disease into chronic or terminal illness.

A Preventive Closing

Early symptom recognition is not paranoia.
It is participation.

Listening to the body, speaking up, and seeking evaluation
are acts of self-respect, not weakness. Cancer thrives on
time and inattention. Prevention thrives on awareness and
courage.

Final Interlude: What I tell my own family

When people learn that I work in cancer, they often ask what I worry about most.

The truth is, I worry less than they expect.

What I tell my own family is not complicated. It is not a list of prohibitions or an obsession with risk. It is a way of paying attention, early, calmly, and consistently.

I tell them that **screening is not fear**. It is simply respect for time. Cancers that are found early often ask little of us. Those found late ask everything.

I tell them to **take vaccines seriously**, especially those that prevent cancer outright. Few medical interventions are so decisive, so generous in their benefit, and so misunderstood.

I remind them that the body does not thrive on extremes. It prefers regular movement, food that resembles what it once was, sleep that follows the night, and days that are not permanently interrupted. None of this needs perfection. Consistency matters more.

I tell them that **alcohol is not harmless**, even when it is ordinary. That tobacco is never worth negotiating with. That sunlight is a gift, but not an entitlement.

I tell them to listen to what persists. Pain that lingers. Bleeding that recurs. Fatigue that does not lift. The body whispers long before it shouts.

I also tell them something that surprises people: that life is not meant to be lived under constant surveillance.

Joy matters. Connection matters. Laughter changes physiology. Isolation leaves marks no scan can detect. Being at peace with oneself is not indulgent, it is stabilising.

I do not tell them they can control everything. No one can. Genetics, chance, and time still have their say. But I do tell them that **risk is not destiny**, and that small, unremarkable choices made over years often matter more than dramatic interventions made too late.

Above all, I tell them this:

Cancer prevention is not about living cautiously. It is about living **attentively**.

Paying attention to the body that carries you.
To the people who depend on you.
To the years you still have.

That, more than anything, is what I tell my own family.

The Moment of Hesitation

There was a moment, long after I had learned the pathways
and memorised the risks, when I hesitated. A test I could
have ordered immediately. A screening I knew I qualified
for. I delayed, not out of ignorance, but out of the quiet
human instinct to postpone certainty. It struck me then that
knowledge does not grant immunity from fear. Even
for neurosurgeons, prevention is not only a scientific act but
an emotional one. We do not avoid information because we
doubt it. We avoid it because it asks us to confront time.

Epilogue

Cancer itself is rarely the final killer.
Metastasis is.

When malignant cells escape their tissue of origin and establish themselves elsewhere, bone, liver, brain, lung, they carry their identity with them. They grow where they do not belong, serve no function, and resist every attempt to reclaim order. Even in the genomic era, metastatic disease remains our greatest challenge.

This is why time matters.

Delay is not neutral. Every postponed symptom, every dismissed signal, grants biology the advantage. What begins silently accumulates momentum. By the time it announces itself, options narrow. Consequences multiply.

Modern life has made attentiveness harder than ever. Communication has thinned. Even within families, illness is minimised, deferred, or quietly ignored. We live in a world saturated with distraction, where attention is monetised and silence is mistaken for health.

Only then do we step back far enough to see the scale of the problem.

Cancer has existed for more than a million years.
Only in recent decades have we begun to understand it
with clarity.

Its devastation still defies language. Cancer is not merely a
disease of cells, but of lives, of families, identities, futures
quietly interrupted. Modern oncology has transformed
what is possible: targeted therapies that block precise
molecular signals, immunotherapies that recruit the
immune system itself, and increasingly refined genetic
classification of disease. Chemotherapy, blunt, imperfect,
and often brutal, remains indispensable, not because it is
ideal, but because we are not yet free of it.

It is a strange moment in human history. Never have we
had greater access to knowledge, yet rarely has life felt so
casually spent. We reward visibility over substance,
applause over contribution, entertainment over endurance.

Women's health remains especially vulnerable to this
neglect. Mothers, partners, caregivers, so often the
structural core of families, are frequently the last to be
asked whether they are nourished, rested, or well. As age
advances and mutations accumulate, vigilance must replace
complacency. **Screening is not fear. It is foresight.**

The strategies outlined in this book are not guarantees.
Cancer is not entirely preventable. Genetics, chance, and
biology still matter. But prevention is not futile. Cancer

does not merely shorten life, it erodes its quality, often long before its end.

Many people believe they were simply unlucky. Sometimes that is true. But often, risk is cumulative, shaped quietly over decades by choices mistaken for habits.

Prevention, at its core, is not radical.

It is movement.
It is food that nourishes rather than inflames.
It is restraint with alcohol, avoidance of tobacco, respect for sleep.
It is vaccination, screening, and attention.

And it is, perhaps most underestimated of all, peace of mind.

Happiness is not naïve. Chronic despair, isolation, and unrelieved stress leave biological traces. To live attentively, connected to others, and at ease with oneself is not indulgence, it is protective.

In the vast universe, on a small planet with molten magma turning endlessly beneath our feet, we are brief visitors. As Theophrastus, successor to Aristotle, once observed:

"Nature has given to deer and to crows a life so long and so useless, and to man only one that is often very short."

If our time is limited, then it deserves care.

Care for the body that carries us.

Care for the mind that interprets the world.

Care for the relationships that give life meaning.

And above all:

Do not surrender these years, few as they are, to the crab.

Appendix

What to Do

This book has asked you to think differently about cancer, not as an unavoidable catastrophe, but as a process that often unfolds quietly, over time.

What follows is not a prescription. It is a way of paying attention.

1. Do not delay what persists

Symptoms that do not resolve deserve investigation. Delay is not neutral. Early attention often determines whether intervention is simple or complex, curative or palliative.

Listening to your body is not anxiety. It is intelligence.

2. Screen on time

Screening exists because many cancers begin silently. Mammography, cervical screening, colonoscopy, skin checks, these are not acts of fear. They are acts of foresight.

When screening works, nothing happens. That is the point.

3. Vaccinate early

Some cancers are preventable in the most literal sense. Vaccines against hepatitis B and human papillomavirus have already saved millions of lives.

Prevention is most powerful before exposure, before symptoms, before the need for courage.

4. Move often

Physical activity does not need to be extreme to be protective. Regular movement regulates metabolism, reduces inflammation, supports immune surveillance, and improves mental health.

The body was not designed for stillness.

5. Eat recognisably

Choose foods that resemble their natural form. Favour plants, whole grains, legumes, fruits, and vegetables. Limit ultra-processed foods, excess sugar, and unnecessary calories.

Nutrition is not about perfection. It is about patterns, sustained over time.

6. Respect sleep

Sleep is not a luxury. It regulates hormones, immune function, DNA repair, and circadian rhythm.

Protect the night. Darkness matters.

7. Use alcohol sparingly and avoid tobacco completely

Alcohol is a carcinogen. Tobacco remains one of the most potent cancer-causing agents ever introduced into human behavior.

There is no safe level of tobacco use. Less alcohol is always better than more.

8. Guard your peace

Chronic stress, isolation, and unresolved despair leave biological traces. Emotional health is not separate from physical health.

Connection, purpose, and contentment are not indulgences. They are protective factors.

9. Share responsibility

Cancer prevention does not belong solely to individuals. It depends on families, communities, clinicians, educators, and policy.

Speak openly. Ask questions. Make prevention visible.

10. Remember what success looks like

The greatest victories in cancer prevention are invisible.

No diagnosis.
No treatment.
No story to tell.

If nothing happens, it has worked.

A Final Word

You do not need to change everything.
You do not need to live in fear.

Small, informed choices, made calmly and repeated over time, can shift risk meaningfully.

Prevention is not control.
It is care.

And care, sustained quietly, is how lives are extended, not dramatically, but deeply.

References

(Organized by Chapter)

Chapter 1 – Cancer: An Ancient Disease in a Modern World

1. Rothschild B, Witzke B, Hershkovitz I. Metastatic cancer in the Jurassic. *Lancet*. 1999;354(9176):398.
2. Odes EJ, Randolph-Quinney PS, Steyn M, et al. Earliest hominin cancer: A 1.7-million-year-old osteosarcoma from South Africa. *S Afr J Sci*. 2016;112(7–8).
3. Zimmerman MR. Evidence of cancer in ancient mummies. In: Aufderheide AC, ed. *The Scientific Study of Mummies*. Cambridge University Press; 2003:373.
4. Feldman M, Hershkovitz I, Sklan E, et al. Detection of a tumor suppressor gene variant predisposing to colorectal cancer in an 18th-century Hungarian mummy. *PLOS ONE*. 2016;11(2):e0147217.
5. Breasted JH. *The Edwin Smith Surgical Papyrus*. University of Chicago Press; 1930.
6. Ebbell B. *The Papyrus Ebers*. Oxford University Press; 1937.
7. Galen. *De temperamentis et de inaequali intemperie libri tres*. Cambridge: John Siberch; 1521.
8. Vesalius A. *De humani corporis fabrica*. Basel; 1543.
9. Paracelsus. *Selected Writings*. Princeton University Press; 1951.
10. Hill J. *Cautions Against the Immoderate Use of Snuff*. London; 1761.
11. Pott P. Cancer scroti. In: *Chirurgical Observations*. London; 1775.
12. Rehn L. Blasengeschwülste bei Fuchsinarbeitern. *Arch Klin Chir*. 1895;50:588–600.
13. Boveri T. Zur Frage der Entstehung maligner Tumoren. Jena; 1914.

Chapter 2 – You Are What You Eat

14. Huttenhower C, Gevers D, Knight R, et al. Structure, function and diversity of the healthy human microbiome. *Nature*. 2012;486:207–214.
15. Allwood AC, Walter MR, Kamber BS, Marshall CP, Burch IW. Stromatolite reef from the Early Archaean era of Australia. *Nature*. 2006;441:714–718.
16. Butterfield NJ, Knoll AH, Swett K. Exceptional preservation of fossils in Neoproterozoic cap carbonates. *Nature*. 1990;344:424–427.
17. Bäckhed F, Ley RE, Sonnenburg JL, Peterson DA, Gordon JI. Host-bacterial mutualism in the human intestine. *Science*. 2005;307:1915–1920.
18. Martin FPJ, Dumas ME, Wang Y, et al. A top-down systems biology view of microbiome–host metabolic interactions. *Mol Syst Biol*. 2007;3:112.
19. Metchnikoff E. *The Prolongation of Life*. London: Heinemann; 1907.

20. Piewngam P, Zheng Y, Nguyen TH, et al. Pathogen elimination by probiotic Bacillus via signaling interference. *Nature*. 2018;562:532–537.

21. Mills JP, Rao K, Young VB. Probiotics for prevention of *Clostridioides difficile* infection. *Curr Opin Gastroenterol*. 2018;34(1):3–10.

22. Link-Amster H, Rochat F, Saudan KY, Mignot O, Aeschlimann JM. Modulation of immune response through fermented milk intake. *FEMS Immunol Med Microbiol*. 1994;10:55–63.

23. Łaniewski P, Barnes D, Goulder A, et al. Linking cervicovaginal immune signatures with microbiome dysbiosis. *Nat Commun*. 2018;9:5127.

24. Verhoeven V, Renard N, Makar A, et al. Probiotics enhance clearance of HPV-related cervical lesions. *Eur J Cancer Prev*. 2013;22(1):46–51.

Chapter 3 – When Life Loses Its Rhythm

25. Damiola F, Le Minh N, Preitner N, et al. Restricted feeding uncouples circadian oscillators. *Genes Dev*. 2000;14:2950–2961.

26. Yang W, Deng Q, Fan W, Wang W, Wang X. Light exposure at night and breast cancer risk. *Eur J Cancer Prev*. 2014;23(4):269–276.

27. Schernhammer ES, Laden F, Speizer FE, et al. Night-shift work and colorectal cancer risk. *JNCI*. 2003;95(11):825–828.

28. Amano H, Fukuda Y, Yokoo T, Yamaoka K. Interleukin-6 levels among shift workers. *J Atheroscler Thromb*. 2018;25(12):1206–1214.

29. McNeely E, Mordukhovich I, Staffa S, et al. Cancer prevalence among flight attendants. *Environ Health*. 2018;17:49.

30. Garaulet M, Gómez-Abellán P. Timing of food intake and obesity. *Physiol Behav*. 2014;134:44–50.

31. Srour B, et al. Circadian nutritional behaviors and cancer risk. *Int J Cancer*. 2018;143:2369–2379.

32. Gibbs J, Ince L, Matthews L, et al. Circadian clock control of inflammation. *Nat Med*. 2014;20:919–926.

Chapter 4 – A Sweet Way to Be Fat: Obesity, Sugar, and Cancer

1. World Health Organization. *Global Database on Body Mass Index: BMI Classification*. WHO; 2017.

2. Spechler SJ. Barrett's esophagus and esophageal adenocarcinoma: pathogenesis, diagnosis, and therapy. *Gastroenterology*. 2013;145(6):1230–1238.

3. Carreras-Torres R, Johansson M, Gaborieau V, et al. The role of obesity, type 2 diabetes, and metabolic factors in pancreatic cancer: A Mendelian randomization study. *J Natl Cancer Inst*. 2017;109(9).

4. Khan FZ, Perumpail RB, Wong RJ, et al. Advances in hepatocellular carcinoma: nonalcoholic steatohepatitis-related hepatocellular carcinoma. *World J Hepatol*. 2015;7:2155–2161.

5. Murphy N, Cross AJ, Abubakar M, et al. Metabolically defined body size phenotypes and colorectal cancer risk. *PLoS Med.* 2016;13:e1001988.

6. Jenab M, Riboli E, Cleveland RJ, et al. Serum C-peptide, IGFBP-1, IGFBP-2 and colorectal cancer risk. *Int J Cancer.* 2007;121:368–376.

7. Key TJ, Appleby PN, Reeves GK, et al. Circulating sex hormones and breast cancer risk. *Br J Cancer.* 2011;105:709–722.

8. Gunter MJ, Hoover DR, Yu H, et al. Insulin, IGF-I, and breast cancer risk. *J Natl Cancer Inst.* 2009;101:48–60.

9. Liao LM, Weinstein SJ, Pollak M, et al. Circulating adipokines and renal cell carcinoma risk. *Carcinogenesis.* 2013;34:109–112.

10. Gamage SMK, Dissabandara L, Lam AK, Gopalan V. Heme iron and colorectal carcinogenesis. *Crit Rev Oncol Hematol.* 2018;126:121–128.

11. Severi G, Morris HA, MacInnis RJ, et al. Circulating steroid hormones and prostate cancer risk. *Cancer Epidemiol Biomarkers Prev.* 2006;15:86–91.

12. Liao LM, et al. Obesity, hypertension, adiponectin and renal cancer risk. *Carcinogenesis.* 2013;34:109–112.

Chapter 5 – Physical Inactivity

13. Friedenreich CM, Neilson HK, Lynch BM. Physical activity and cancer prevention: mechanisms and evidence. *Eur J Cancer.* 2010;46:2593–2604.

14. Moore SC, Lee IM, Weiderpass E, et al. Leisure-time physical activity and cancer risk in 1.44 million adults. *JAMA Intern Med.* 2016;176:816–825.

15. Aune D, Chan DSM, Lau R, et al. Physical activity and cancer risk: dose–response meta-analysis. *BMJ.* 2011;343:d6617.

16. Gibbs J, Ince L, Matthews L, et al. Circadian clock regulation of inflammation and glucocorticoid action. *Nat Med.* 2014;20:919–926.

17. Friedenreich CM. Physical activity and immune function. *Cancer Epidemiol Biomarkers Prev.* 2001;10:287–293.

18. Meadows GG, Zhang H. Effects of alcohol and inactivity on tumor growth and immune surveillance. *Alcohol Res.* 2015;37:311–322.

19. Kinney JP, Long CS, Geller AC. The ultraviolet index as a public health tool. *Dermatol Online J.* 2000;6(1).

20. Dennis LK, Vanbeek MJ, Freeman LEB, et al. Childhood sunburns and melanoma risk. *Ann Epidemiol.* 2008;18:614–627.

21. Sport England. *Active Lives Adult Survey Report 2016–2017.*

22. Scottish Government. *Scottish Health Survey 2016.*

23. Welsh Government. *National Survey for Wales 2016–2017.*

24. Northern Ireland Statistics and Research Agency. *Health Survey Northern Ireland 2016–2017.*

25. Srour B, et al. Circadian nutritional behaviors and cancer risk. *Int J Cancer*. 2018;143:2369–2379.

26. Garaulet M, Gómez-Abellán P. Timing of food intake and obesity. *Physiol Behav*. 2014;134:44–50.

27. Damiola F, Le Minh N, Preitner N, et al. Feeding schedules uncouple circadian oscillators. *Genes Dev*. 2000;14:2950–2961.

28. Yatsuya H, Tsugane S. What constitutes healthiness of the Japanese diet (Washoku)?. *Eur J Clin Nutr*. 2021.

29. Wei Y, Lv J, Guo Y, et al. Soy intake and breast cancer risk: prospective cohort study. *Eur J Epidemiol*. 2020;35:567–578.

30. Aune D, Chan DSM, Lau R, et al. Dietary fiber, whole grains, and colorectal cancer. *BMJ*. 2011;343:d6617.

31. Fung TT, Chiuve SE, Willett WC, et al. Fruit and vegetable intake and ER-negative breast cancer. *Breast Cancer Res Treat*. 2013;138:925–930.

32. Zhang X, et al. Calcium intake and colorectal cancer risk. *Int J Cancer*. 2016;139:2232–2242.

33. Fahey JW, Talalay P, Kensler TW. Sulforaphane and cancer prevention. *Proc Natl Acad Sci USA*. 2002;99:7610–7615.

34. Mazidi M, Ferns G, Banach M. Tomato and lycopene intake and cancer mortality. *Public Health Nutr*. 2020;23:1569–1575.

35. Jin Z, Wu M, Han R, et al. Raw garlic consumption and lung cancer risk. *Cancer Prev Res*. 2013;6:711–718.

36. Chen Y, Nakanishi M, Rosenberg DW. Walnuts, gut microbiota, and colon cancer prevention. *Cancer Prev Res*. 2019;13:15–24.

Chapter 7 – Tobacco: An Everlasting Pandemic

1. Doll R, Hill AB. Smoking and carcinoma of the lung: preliminary report. *BMJ*. 1950;2:739–748.

2. Doll R, Peto R, Wheatley K, Gray R, Sutherland I. Mortality in relation to smoking: 40 years' observations on male British doctors. *BMJ*. 1994;309:901–911.

3. Doll R, Peto R, Boreham J, Sutherland I. Mortality in relation to smoking: 50 years' observations on male British doctors. *BMJ*. 2004;328:1519.

4. US Surgeon General. *The Health Consequences of Smoking—50 Years of Progress*. US Department of Health and Human Services; 2014.

5. Song MA, Benowitz NL, Berman M, et al. Cigarette filter ventilation and increasing rates of lung adenocarcinoma. *J Natl Cancer Inst*. 2017;109(12).

6. Pott P. Chirurgical observations relative to the cancer of the scrotum. London: Hawes, Clarke & Collins; 1775.

7. Rehn L. Bladder tumors in fuchsin workers. *Arch Klin Chir*. 1895;50:588–600.

8. World Health Organization. *WHO Report on the Global Tobacco Epidemic*. WHO; 2021.

9. Hecht SS. Tobacco smoke carcinogens and lung cancer. *J Natl Cancer Inst*. 1999;91:1194–1210.

10. Benowitz NL. Nicotine addiction. *N Engl J Med*. 2010;362:2295–2303.

11. Glantz SA, Slade J, Bero LA, Hanauer P, Barnes DE. The cigarette papers. *JAMA*. 1996;275:248–253.

12. Mills SD. Project HIPPO: tobacco industry internal research on nicotine addiction. *Tob Control*. 1998;7:92–101.

Chapter 8 – Alcohol: A Toast to Cancer

13. International Agency for Research on Cancer. Alcohol consumption and ethyl carbamate. *IARC Monographs*. Vol 96. 2010.

14. Seitz HK, Stickel F. Acetaldehyde as an underestimated risk factor for cancer development. *Genes Nutr*. 2010;5:121–128.

15. Boffetta P, Hashibe M. Alcohol and cancer. *Lancet Oncol*. 2006;7:149–156.

16. Ahrens W, Pohlabeln H, Foraita R, et al. Oral health, mouthwash use, and aerodigestive cancers. *Oral Oncol*. 2014;50:616–625.

17. Boffetta P, Hayes RB, Sartori S, et al. Mouthwash use and head and neck cancer. *Eur J Cancer Prev*. 2016;25:344–348.

18. Meadows GG, Zhang H. Effects of alcohol on tumor growth, metastasis, and immune response. *Alcohol Res*. 2015;37:311–322.

19. Scoccianti C, Lauby-Secretan B, Bello PY, Chajes V, Romieu I. Alcohol consumption and cancer risk. *Lancet Oncol*. 2014;15:e142–e150.

20. Chen WY, Rosner B, Hankinson SE, Colditz GA, Willett WC. Moderate alcohol consumption and breast cancer risk. *JAMA*. 2011;306:1884–1890.

21. World Health Organization. *Global Status Report on Alcohol and Health*. WHO; 2018.

Chapter 9 – A Beautiful Mind: Stress, Biology, and Cancer

22. Galen. *De temperamentis*. Cambridge: John Siberch; 1521.

23. Paget J. *Lectures on Surgical Pathology*. London: Longmans; 1863.

24. Walshe WH. *The Nature and Treatment of Cancer*. London: Taylor & Walton; 1846.

25. Snow HL. *Cancer and the Cancer Process*. London: J & A Churchill; 1893.

26. Peller S. Cancer and its relation to pregnancy, delivery, and marital status. *Surg Gynecol Obstet*. 1940;71:1–8.

27. Butler B. Hypnosis in the care of the cancer patient. *Cancer*. 1954;7:1–14.

28. LeShan L. Some recurrent life history patterns observed in patients with malignant disease. *J Nerv Ment Dis*. 1956;124:460–465.

29. Orbach CE, Sutherland AM, Bozeman MF. Psychological impact of cancer and its treatment. *Cancer*. 1955;8:20–28.

30. Cohen S, Janicki-Deverts D, Miller GE. Psychological stress and disease. *JAMA*. 2007;298:1685–1687.

31. Epel ES, Blackburn EH, Lin J, et al. Accelerated telomere shortening in response to life stress. *Proc Natl Acad Sci USA*. 2004;101:17312–17315.

32. Antoni MH, Lutgendorf SK, Cole SW, et al. The influence of stress and social support on cancer biology. *Nat Rev Cancer*. 2006;6:240–248.

33. Zhang B, et al. Hyperactivation of sympathetic nerves drives depletion of melanocyte stem cells. *Nature*. 2020;577:676–681.

34. Senga SS, Grose RP. Hallmarks of cancer—the new testament. *Open Biol*. 2021;11:200358.

Chapter 10 – Precision Prevention of Breast Cancer

1. Cancer Research UK. *Breast cancer incidence by age*. CRUK; latest update.

2. Collaborative Group on Hormonal Factors in Breast Cancer. Menarche, menopause, and breast cancer risk. *Lancet Oncol*. 2012;13:1141–1151.

3. Sisti JS, et al. Reproductive risk factors and molecular subtypes of breast cancer. *Int J Cancer*. 2016;138:2346–2356.

4. Albrektsen G, Heuch I, Hansen S, Kvale G. Breast cancer risk by age at birth and parity. *Br J Cancer*. 2005;92:167–175.

5. MacMahon B, et al. Age at first birth and breast cancer risk. *Bull WHO*. 1970;43:209–221.

6. Lambe M, et al. Transient increase in breast cancer risk after childbirth. *N Engl J Med*. 1994;331:5–9.

7. Collaborative Group on Breastfeeding and Breast Cancer. Breastfeeding and breast cancer risk. *Lancet*. 2002;360:187–195.

8. Key TJ, et al. Circulating sex hormones and breast cancer risk. *Br J Cancer*. 2011;105:709–722.

9. Boynton-Jarrett R, et al. Gestational weight gain and daughter's age at menarche. *J Womens Health*. 2011;20:1193–1200.

10. Wei Y, et al. Soy intake and breast cancer risk: China Kadoorie Biobank. *Eur J Epidemiol*. 2020;35:567–578.

11. McKenzie F, et al. Healthy lifestyle and breast cancer risk (EPIC). *Int J Cancer*. 2015;136:2640–2648.

12. US Preventive Services Task Force. BRCA-related cancer risk assessment and testing. *JAMA*. 2019;322:652–665.

13. Antoniou A, et al. Breast and ovarian cancer risks in BRCA1/2 mutation carriers. *Am J Hum Genet*. 2003;72:1117–1130.

Chapter 11 – Precision Prevention of Colorectal Cancer

14. International Agency for Research on Cancer. *Globocan 2018: Colorectal Cancer*. IARC.
15. Aune D, et al. Dietary fibre, whole grains, and colorectal cancer risk. *BMJ*. 2011;343:d6617.
16. Zhang X, et al. Calcium intake and colorectal cancer risk. *Int J Cancer*. 2016;139:2232–2242.
17. Gamage SMK, et al. Role of heme iron in colorectal carcinogenesis. *Crit Rev Oncol Hematol*. 2018;126:121–128.
18. Moore SC, et al. Physical activity and cancer risk in 1.44 million adults. *JAMA Intern Med*. 2016;176:816–825.
19. Patel SG, Ahnen DJ. Familial colon cancer syndromes. *Curr Gastroenterol Rep*. 2012;14:428–438.
20. Lynch HT, de la Chapelle A. Hereditary colorectal cancer. *N Engl J Med*. 2003;348:919–932.
21. Jasperson KW, et al. Familial adenomatous polyposis. *Gastroenterology*. 2010;138:2044–2058.
22. Winawer SJ, et al. Colorectal cancer screening and polyp removal. *N Engl J Med*. 1993;329:1977–1981.
23. Murphy N, et al. Metabolic body size phenotypes and colorectal cancer. *PLoS Med*. 2016;13:e1001988.
24. Odes EJ, et al. Earliest hominin cancer. *S Afr J Sci*. 2016;112:7–8.

Chapter 12 – Precision Prevention of Melanoma

25. International Agency for Research on Cancer. *Solar and ultraviolet radiation*. IARC Monographs Vol 100D; 2012.
26. Mitra D, et al. UV-independent melanoma in red-hair phenotype. *Nature*. 2012;491:449–453.
27. Dennis LK, et al. Sunburns and melanoma risk: meta-analysis. *Ann Epidemiol*. 2008;18:614–627.
28. Wehner MR, et al. Indoor tanning and skin cancer. *BMJ*. 2012;345:e5909.
29. Kinney JP, et al. The ultraviolet index as a public health tool. *Dermatol Online J*. 2000;6:1.

30. Quatresooz P, et al. Photoaging under sunbeds. *Skin Res Technol*. 2011;17:309–313.

31. Lo JA, Fisher DE. UV carcinogenesis and melanoma therapeutics. *Science*. 2014;346:945–949.

32. Zhang B, et al. Stress-induced depletion of melanocyte stem cells. *Nature*. 2020;577:676–681.

33. Cooperstone JL, et al. Tomatoes protect against UV-induced skin carcinogenesis. *Sci Rep*. 2017;7:5106.

34. Young AJ. Photoprotective role of carotenoids in plants. *Physiol Plant*. 1991;83:702–708.

35. Wheeler BW, et al. Radon exposure and skin cancer risk. *Epidemiology*. 2012;23:44–52.

Chapter 13 – Precision Prevention of Liver Cancer

1. International Agency for Research on Cancer. *Globocan 2018: Liver Cancer*. IARC.

2. World Health Organization. *Global Health Sector Strategy on Viral Hepatitis 2016–2021*. WHO; 2016.

3. Chang MH, et al. Universal hepatitis B vaccination and reduction of hepatocellular carcinoma. *N Engl J Med*. 1997;336:1855–1859.

4. Chen DS. Hepatitis B vaccination: the key to eliminating hepatocellular carcinoma. *J Hepatol*. 2009;50:805–816.

5. Khan FZ, et al. Nonalcoholic steatohepatitis-related hepatocellular carcinoma. *World J Hepatol*. 2015;7:2155–2166.

6. Perz JF, et al. Contribution of hepatitis B and C infections to liver cancer worldwide. *J Hepatol*. 2006;45:529–538.

7. World Health Organization. *Hepatitis C Fact Sheet*. WHO; latest update.

8. Blount WP. Turkey "X" disease. *J Br Turkey Fed*. 1961;9:55–58.

9. Kensler TW, Roebuck BD, Wogan GN, Groopman JD. Aflatoxin: a 50-year odyssey. *Toxicol Sci*. 2011;120(Suppl 1):S28–S48.

10. Groopman JD, Kensler TW. Role of aflatoxin in liver cancer. *Gastroenterology*. 2005;127:S52–S60.

11. International Agency for Research on Cancer. *Aflatoxins*. IARC Monographs Vol 100F; 2012.

12. Seitz HK, Stickel F. Acetaldehyde as a risk factor for liver cancer. *Genes Nutr*. 2010;5:121–128.

Chapter 14 – Precision Prevention of Cervical Cancer

13. International Agency for Research on Cancer. *Human papillomaviruses*. IARC Monographs Vol 100B; 2012.

14. zur Hausen H. Papillomaviruses and cancer. *N Engl J Med.* 2009;361:2699–2701.

15. Howley PM, et al. Papillomavirus E6 and E7 oncogenes. *Cold Spring Harb Perspect Med.* 2012;2:a012526.

16. Moody CA, Laimins LA. Human papillomavirus oncogenes. *Nat Rev Cancer.* 2010;10:550–560.

17. Papanicolaou GN, Traut HF. Diagnosis of uterine cancer by the vaginal smear. *Am J Obstet Gynecol.* 1941;42:193–206.

18. Ayre JE. Selective cytology smear for diagnosis of cervical cancer. *J Obstet Gynaecol Br Emp.* 1947;54:426–433.

19. Frazer IH. Development of the HPV vaccine. *Nat Rev Immunol.* 2004;4:46–54.

20. Schiller JT, Lowy DR. Prophylactic HPV vaccines. *J Clin Invest.* 2012;122:438–444.

21. Harper DM, et al. Efficacy of HPV vaccines against cervical neoplasia. *Lancet.* 2004;364:1757–1765.

22. Verhoeven V, et al. Probiotics enhance clearance of HPV-related lesions. *Eur J Cancer Prev.* 2013;22:46–51.

23. NHS England. *Cervical Screening Programme.* Latest guidelines.

Chapter 15 – Precision Prevention of Prostate Cancer

24. Ferlay J, et al. Global cancer statistics: Prostate cancer. *CA Cancer J Clin.* 2018;68:394–424.

25. Severi G, et al. Circulating steroid hormones and prostate cancer risk. *Cancer Epidemiol Biomarkers Prev.* 2006;15:86–91.

26. Rider JR, et al. Ejaculation frequency and prostate cancer risk. *Eur Urol.* 2016;70:974–982.

27. Giovannucci E. Epidemiologic characteristics of prostate cancer. *Cancer.* 2002;94:186–190.

28. Platz EA, De Marzo AM. Prostate inflammation and carcinogenesis. *Nat Rev Cancer.* 2004;4:256–267.

29. Hayes RB, et al. Circumcision and prostate cancer risk. *Cancer Epidemiol Biomarkers Prev.* 2000;9:985–990.

30. Harvard T.H. Chan School of Public Health. *Prostate Cancer Prevention Overview.*

31. Rider JR, et al. Lifestyle factors and prostate cancer progression. *J Natl Cancer Inst.* 2015;107:djv176.

Chapter 16 – Precision Prevention: Environmental Risk Factors

1. International Agency for Research on Cancer. *Agents Classified by the IARC Monographs.* IARC.

2. Darby S, et al. Residential radon and lung cancer. *Scand J Work Environ Health.* 2006;32(Suppl 1):1–83.

3. Krewski D, et al. Radon and lung cancer risk in North America. *J Toxicol Environ Health A*. 2006;69:533–597.

4. Gray A, Read S, McGale P, Darby S. Lung cancer deaths from indoor radon and cost-effectiveness of control policies. *BMJ*. 2009;338:a3110.

5. Lantz PM, Mendez D, Philbert MA. Radon, smoking, and lung cancer. *Am J Public Health*. 2013;103:443–447.

6. Raaschou-Nielsen O. Indoor radon and childhood leukemia. *Radiat Prot Dosimetry*. 2008;132:175–181.

7. Ludwig Rehn. Bladder tumors in dye workers. *Arch Klin Chir*. 1895;50:588–600.

8. Grandjean P, et al. Perfluorinated compounds and vaccine antibody response. *J Immunotoxicol*. 2017;14:188–195.

9. EPA. *Lifetime Health Advisories for PFOS and PFOA*. US Environmental Protection Agency; 2016.

10. Peng C, et al. Low-dose radon exposure and breast tumor gene expression. *BMC Cancer*. 2020;20:695.

11. Wang Z, et al. Arsenic and benzo(a)pyrene co-exposure synergizes lung tumorigenesis. *Cancer Prev Res*. 2020.

12. Wheeler BW, et al. Radon and skin cancer in southwest England. *Epidemiology*. 2012;23:44–52.

13. IARC. *Outdoor air pollution*. IARC Monographs Vol 109; 2016.

Chapter 17 – Precision Prevention: Infections Beyond HPV and Hepatitis

1. International Agency for Research on Cancer. *Biological Agents*. IARC Monographs Vol 100B; 2012.

2. Epstein MA, Achong BG, Barr YM. Virus particles in Burkitt's lymphoma. *Lancet*. 1964;1:702–703.

3. Young LS, Rickinson AB. Epstein–Barr virus: 40 years on. *Nat Rev Cancer*. 2004;4:757–768.

4. Howley PM, Lowy DR. Papillomaviruses and cancer. *J Clin Invest*. 2001;108:145–149.

5. Chang Y, Moore PS. Merkel cell polyomavirus and Merkel cell carcinoma. *J Virol*. 2012;86:8579–8587.

6. Parsonnet J, et al. Helicobacter pylori and gastric carcinoma. *N Engl J Med*. 1991;325:1127–1131.

7. Fahey JW, et al. Sulforaphane and Helicobacter pylori. *PNAS*. 2002;99:7610–7615.

8. Li W, et al. Garlic supplementation and gastric cancer. *BMJ*. 2019;366:l5016.

9. Verdrengh M, et al. Genistein inhibits Helicobacter pylori. *Microbes Infect*. 2004;6:86–92.

10. Plummer M, et al. Global burden of cancers attributable to infection. *Lancet Glob Health*. 2016;4:e609–e616.

11. zur Hausen H. Infections causing human cancer. *Int J Cancer*. 2009;125:165–170.

12. IARC. *Schistosoma haematobium*. IARC Monographs Vol 100B; 2012.

13. WHO. *Global Health Estimates: Cancer Attributable to Infection*.

Chapter 18 – Early Symptoms People Ignore

(This chapter is evidence-guided but clinically grounded; references emphasise delay, stage migration, and outcomes.)

1. Richards MA, et al. Influence of delay on survival in cancer. *Lancet*. 1999;353:1119–1126.

2. Neal RD, et al. Is diagnosis delay associated with cancer survival? *Br J Cancer*. 2015;112:S92–S107.

3. Hiom SC. Diagnosing cancer earlier: why it matters. *Br J Cancer*. 2015;112:S1–S5.

4. Lyratzopoulos G, et al. Variation in diagnostic delay by cancer type. *Lancet Oncol*. 2012;13:353–365.

5. Cancer Research UK. *Early Diagnosis Evidence Base*.

6. Rubin G, et al. Symptoms and signs of cancer. *Lancet*. 2015;385:223–234.

7. Macleod U, et al. Risk of cancer in patients with common symptoms. *Br J Gen Pract*. 2009;59:e308–e315.

8. Hamilton W. Cancer diagnosis in primary care. *BMJ*. 2010;340:c1260.

9. Whitaker KL, et al. Patient delay in cancer presentation. *Psychooncology*. 2015;24:1–10.

10. Emery JD, et al. The role of primary care in early cancer detection. *Lancet Oncol*. 2014;15:e493–e505.

11. Walter FM, et al. Symptoms and early cancer diagnosis. *Nat Rev Clin Oncol*. 2012;9:541–550.

www.ingramcontent.com/pod-product-compliance
Lightning Source LLC
Chambersburg PA
CBHW041304210326
41598CB00005B/22